What others are saying ab

"Miracles" is a powerful word for anyone who has had a stroke. Robinson's tale of a medical treatment that can make the impossible possible --reverse the impairments of strokes -- is a must read for healthcare providers and families of stroke patients. Well researched and based on her father's case history it describes a revolutionary, simple and non-invasive treatment that offers hope and delivers recovery.

Nancy Butler-Ross
Miami Herald Columnist/Author

I was introduced to the full-force Woody Robinson thirty-five years ago. Years later, I witnessed close-up his painful post-stroke decline and increasing desperation. His recuperation was, indeed, the "miracle" Robin Robinson describes so accurately in her attention-grabbing book. Should I ever have a stroke or be diagnosed with another cardio-vascular-related disease, I'd follow in Woody's footsteps instantly.

Marcia Schnedler
Nationally Syndicated Columnist in Travel for 50-Plus Americans

"It reads like I am talking over a coffee table with the author."

Esme Codell
Educating Esme, How to Get Your Child to Love Reading

"I never imagined that a book about reversing stroke damage could be a page turner; but Robin Robinson's book is that".

Rosalind Brackenbury
Solares Hill, The Key West Citizen

What others are saying about Dr. Hammesfahr's Revolutionary Therapy for Stroke Recovery

"Dr. Hammesfahr's pioneering work has resulted in fundamental change, not only in the understanding of closed head injury and stroke, but also in the prognosis for closed head injury and stroke in patients."

Michael Bilirakis, U. S. House of Representatives, Chairman of the Subcommittee on Health and Environment

"Dr. William M. Hammesfahr has through exceptional service, humanitarian efforts and notable achievement been a leader in his field for the advancement of medical technology that has benefited those police officers who's lives and physical abilities have been drastically changed and left facing adversity without hope of a productive future, from injuries sustained while in the service to their communities."

GDM Munson III National Vice President, National Association of Police American Federations of Police

"I admit I came to Clearwater with a certain degree of skepticism. After having the opportunity to observe you and independently interview your patients, I have modified my opinion. I now fully understand the rationale behind your treatment regimen. I think this offers a promising pharmaceutical intervention for individuals with a host of neurologic disorders."

Edward Dabrowski, M.D. Chief, Division of Physical Medicine and Rehabilitation Wayne State University

"I am a physician and a stroke survivor. I have found this therapy to be disciplined, non-experimental and successful."

William C. Flanagan, Jr., M.D.
St. Francis Medical Park
Columbus, GA

"I must say that I am unduly impressed. This nouveau approach is certainly exciting as it appears to help the patient with 'seemingly permanent disabilities.' I plan to incorporate this method of treating stroke patients in my practice, and teaching my Residents this method. I hope that I will be able to offer my patients more than I have been able to do in the past."

David B. Levine, D.P.M., D.O., F.A.C.F.P
Department of Family Medicine
Nova Southeastern University

"You should be especially proud of your skills and the humanitarian compassion you display towards others. You are a rare commodity in our society and one which others should recognize and follow."

Peter D. Blume
President/Chief Executive Officer
Vietnam Veterans of America, Inc.

Our congratulations on your outstanding achievement and our best wishes for your continued progress in the field of brain injury.

Elynor Kazuk
Executive Director
Brain Injury Association of Florida, Inc.

Patient's Comments

"Dr. Hammesfahr has successfully changed the course of countless "ruined" lives.

Jerome Jay Solow, DDS

"By the end of the first week Lena was able to raise her right arm to the level of her head. She, on occasion, would speak in complete sentences."

John Gore

"Vic has actually been able to do 210 bench presses. Not bad for a man who came to Dr. Hammesfahr unable to hold a piece of paper."

The Frantz Family

"You not only saved my life you gave it back to me."

Tony Twist

"Larry continues to surprise us all in recovery from his stroke. He has been receiving treatment from Dr. Hammesfahr with remarkable results."

Anita Senko

"After twelve years of being on a plateau with no real expectation of change, change has been happening! This year has been a signal year for Meg. She is now standing by herself in our pool for ten minute periods. We are so proud of her renewed sense of balance, her new ability to stand without her knees collapsing, and her new sense of self which you can see on her face. She loves being able to stand. She can hold her balance while being helped to walk, and go as much as twelve feet."

Mike and Judith Tippett

Peeling the Onion: Reversing the Ravages of Stroke

A Father/Daughter Journey Through a Revolutionary Medical Treatment for Stroke

BY ROBIN ROBINSON

Introduction by
WILLIAM M. HAMMESFAHR, M.D.
1999 Nobel Prize Nominee

SORA Publishing – Key West, Florida
Published by SORA Publishing
1800 Atlantic Boulevard, A-405
Key West, Florida 33040-5708 USA
sorapublishing@comcast.net

Internet Orders from www.sorapublishing.com

ISBN, print edition   0-9765756-1-2

The Library of Congress Cataloging-in-Publication Data
Robinson, Robin.
Peeling the onion: reversing the ravages of stroke/ a father/daughter journey through a breakthrough treatment for stroke / Robin Robinson
2nd Edition
Library of Congress Control Number – 2005900238

SAN 256-4157

To my mother and father, both disabled by stroke

"But those who have hope and faith will renew their strength

They will soar on wings like eagles.

They will run and not grow weary.

They will walk and not be faint."

    -Isaiah 40:26-31

Contents

About the Author
Introduction by William Hammesfahr, MD

About the Author

Robin Robinson has written for newspapers since the early 1960's. She wrote a weekly bicycle column for the *Chicago Daily News* called "Ride On." Shortly after that she began a weekly column for them called "Parent and Child Together." It was syndicated by Princeton Features and ran for ten years in more than one hundred newspapers as "Robin's World," illustrated by Kay Chorao. Since then she has written travel stories for the *Chicago Sun Times* and other media. She taught high school Advanced Placement writing courses and a four-year Theater Major program for thirty years. She recently retired.

About the Doctor

William Hammesfahr, M.D., is a graduate of Northwestern University's Honors Program in Medical Education. He did his residency at The College of Virginia in neurology and neurosurgery and is Board Certified in Neurology and Pain Management. In 1989 he founded the Hammesfahr Neurological Institute in Clearwater, Florida.

He is an examiner for Social Security in the State of Florida and a reviewer of the Peer Review Board for Grant Funding by the U.S. Department of Education with Special Expertise in credentialing for Neurology, Neurosurgery, and Disability Rehabilitation. He was named Reviewer and Chief Reviewer.

He received commendations and recognition for his work with the following organizations: Disabled Police Veterans Assoc., National Stroke Assoc., Brain Injury Assoc., Vietnam Veterans of America, American Police Hall of Fame, and the State of Florida Department of Labor and Employment Security, Office of Disability Determinations.

Introduction
By William Hammesfahr, MD

Miracles happen every day at the Hammesfahr Neurological Institute in Clearwater, Florida.

Of course, they are not really miracles, but events that seem miraculous. Patients with severely debilitating diseases they had thought incurable suddenly discover that they can get better, after all. They rise up from wheelchairs and walk. They regain the use of paralyzed arms and hands. Their minds, their memories and the sparkles in their eyes return. They speak and laugh and sing again. They realize, with tears of joy, that they will continue to improve.

All doctors are fortunate because they get to help people, but I have been especially blessed. First, I was privileged to develop a treatment with the potential to help so many people with such a wide range of afflictions. And then, a wonderful writer came to our Institute to tell our story.

Robin Robinson brought her father to the Hammesfahr Neurological Institute seeking treatment for a serious stroke he'd had eight years earlier in hopes that he would improve. She kept a daily journal of their experiences during the three weeks they were here, and also recorded the experiences of other patients and caregivers who were here about the hope and courage of families and patients who do not give up after being struck by a catastrophic medical disaster. It is about prayers being answered. It also is the story of an amazing medical breakthrough.

In the simplest terms, our therapy uses common FDA approved vasodilators and extensive ultrasound testing to establish a dose of medications unique to each individual, which opens their damaged and constricted blood vessels. This procedure allows blood to flow into parts of the brain that previously received an inadequate supply. When the blood begins to flow back into the brain, the brain heals itself.

Severe narrowing of the blood vessels is found in many previously untreatable neurological diseases. These diseases read like an encyclopedia of chronic neurological disorders: whiplash, brain injury, concussion, post concussion, spinal cord injuries, migraine, stroke, cerebral palsy, balance problems, memory loss, encephalitis, meningitis, West Nile virus, post polio disease, dyslexia, learning disabilities, emotionally disturbed behavior, attention deficit disorder, attention deficit hyperactive disorder, autism, childhood aphasia, Tourette's syndrome, Parkinson's, seizures, epilepsy, Lou Gehrig's disease (ALS), multiple sclerosis, macular degeneration, some arthritic diseases, some Alzheimer's, diabetic eye and nerve loss, Lupus neurological problems, the chemical attack on the body by itself, psychosis, schizophrenia, and others. All these conditions have in common a fluctuating neurological or cognitive state, and all have the potential to be alleviated by increasing the flow of blood to the brain.

We are no longer at the birth of a new age in the treatment of brain injury, stroke and other vascular diseases; we have grown to adolescence.

Now we know. It's the blood vessels that matter.

We are no longer at the birth of a new age in the treatment of brain injury, stroke and other vascular diseases; we have grown to adolescence.

Now we know. It's the blood vessels that matter.

I am grateful to have found a way to treat so many diseases, to have had that eureka moment when our understanding of these diseases was raised to a whole new level. Thanks in no small part to Robin Robinson, who brought her father and her talent to Druid Road, many others will come to understand it, too.

This is Robin's story of a typical stroke patient, her father, going though the process of recovery using our therapy. You will find comments about our experience with patients at the Hammesfahr Neurological Institute interlaced with hers as she tells this compelling tale.

We thank God for this chance to help.

William Hammesfahr, M.D.
Clearwater, Florida

1
Flights
August

"6A and B," Steve directed as we walked down the narrow aisle in the 747.

"Excellent! We're on the bulkhead," I said. We had a good three feet of space between the seats and the wall separating the compartments. I wrapped my feet in the gray airline blanket, stuffed the pillow behind my right elbow, closed my seat belt, and reached for the airline magazine. Up front, the steward asked the passengers whether they would like drinks before take-off. Steve clicked his seat belt shut. There was a steady buzz from the overhead light fixture and a whoosh from the air vent. I began leafing through the pages looking for a travel story or a good joke.

This was a four-hour flight from LA to Chicago. Although United tends to fill it with food and movies, I knew in my skeptical mind that it was just as possible that the flight would be delayed on the runway and would take six or seven hours. I was half way through a real page-turner, Jack Whyte's novel, "The Skystone," and I didn't want to finish it before we got home. My son, Rollins, had landed his first important job and bought me the book to celebrate. I wanted it fresh in my mind when I talked to him. I paged through the magazine articles about how to pack a suitcase and ads about watches with your company logo on them. Then I saw, in the far right hand corner of the page, the ad.

"PARALYZED FROM A STROKE FOR 4 YEARS, RECOVERED IN 4 MONTHS"

There was a picture of Ron Clark in sunglasses, on a ladder, painting a house. The ad went on.

"Using a new therapy (patent pending) developed by W. Hammesfahr, MD, and the Hammesfahr Neurological Institute, patients are experiencing a high level of recovery. In a peer-reviewed study, 80% of our patients from around the world had major recovery."

My cynical, suspicious mind began to work. Dr. William Hammesfahr. Who is this man? How could he know what no one else in the medical field knows? The press is constantly telling the public horror stories about alternative medicines that don't work. Still, people flock to use over the counter herbs and see homeopathic doctors. Alternative medicine is big business in this country. There are many stories about people who regain health after illness attributed to the 'strength' of the patient or 'spontaneous remission' or 'a miracle.' What kind of therapy could Dr. William Hammesfahr be using? This Dr. Hammesfahr sounded too good to be true.

It seemed like a tabloid story, flamboyant, ridiculous. Then I thought of my father sitting in his big recliner chair that he got out of less and less. Some nights he chose to sleep in it instead of going to bed. He had been felled by a stroke eight years earlier. Bleeding inside his skull a year later had led to further complications.

I remembered sitting with my mother by his hospital bed in Springfield, Illinois, listening to him respond with a slow negative shake of his massive head to simple questions about the place he was born and the year he fell in love. Tears ran down my cheeks, unnoticed by him, mourning the lost mind that, as an educational psychologist, had guided so many young people through their terrors in life. Now the terror was in his own pale blue eyes as he realized that he could not remember.

Shared memories are like secrets between people, more precious when private and infinitely sad when there is no one left to share them. Now, I was the only one to remember the long walk in the woods when my father first explained the ins and outs of sex to a very attentive eleven-year-old. The only one to remember learning the square roots of numbers up to twelve. I never needed this information, but the hours spent learning it during lunches in my father's empty classroom was a sweet memory. I remember, and I may remember it incorrectly, but he didn't remember at all.

My mother believed that she would live as long as someone remembered her. Her children and grandchildren would carry her stories with them and they would be retold from generation to generation, giving our family a history. I would remember that Duke and Duchess, two white oxen, had pulled the cart that brought my farming great-great grandfather to Nebraska. I would remember the sod house that he covered in wood as the farm prospered. I would remember that mother taught in a one-room schoolhouse isolated far out on the Nebraska prairie when she was only sixteen years old. I would remember and I would tell my children. They would remember.

My father gradually recovered his thoughts and some of his memories, but he lost the use of his right hand and he had a difficult time walking two blocks, even with his cane. After six months of rehabilitation he was told he would have no more recovery. That he always would be crippled in his right arm and unable to use his right hand. That his arm always would hurt. That he always would walk with great pain, and a pronounced limp. That he never would bend his knee to take a step, or flex his ankle or his toes. That he always would have difficulty thinking of the right word and that his mind always would be muddled. That he always would be unable to read more than a paragraph without losing focus. That he always would be without his sense of taste and his sense of smell. Always, he would live this way. Unless, of course, he had another stroke, as forty percent of stroke victims do within five years. If he had another stroke, he would get worse.

Always.

Always is a powerful word.

The ad cited a second example, that of an assistant head nurse who suffered a sudden stroke. After two months, she could not speak in understandable sentences. Her words no longer connected with her ideas. She was going to resign from her job the following week and go on disability. Instead, she went to the Hammesfahr Neurological Institute. Within the week, she regained her ability to communicate. Instead of a frustrating life desperately trying to make herself understood, she was able to return to work full time in that one week.

What kind of crazy miracle was that? I daydreamed about how her family members must have felt seeing their loved one recover so quickly from a condition that could have made them caretakers for the rest of her life. I imagined her first intelligible words in the kitchen where her daughter was making eggs for breakfast. I could see the whole family stop what they were doing, not moving for fear the moment would disappear. Her husband is speaking softly, afraid that a loud noise would scramble her brain cells again.

"You said a sentence."

"Yes, I did."

The joy! The glorious joy that the family must have felt!

My eyes filled up with tears and I couldn't read the copy in the ad any more. I wiped the tears away with my fingers and let out a shaky breath. It could happen to us. This could be our family. Dr. Hammesfahr could have my father whole again in a week's time. Then I remembered that this woman had had the stroke just two months before. It was fresh and ready for a response. Her case was special. My father's stroke was eight years old. This treatment probably would not work for more difficult cases, like Dad's. I looked at the ad again. What kind of a doctor advertises in an airline magazine? Doesn't this magazine have any standards? Do they let any crackpot with money put ads in their magazine? Surely the magazine or the medical profession has some quality control. I tried to argue each side of the question. If I were Dr. Hammesfahr and I knew this wonderful way to cure stroke victims, how would I let people know? Stroke victims don't read medical journals. I had seen rows of wheelchairs routinely await invalid Northern snowbirds at the Miami airport. Where better to advertise than in an airline magazine?

The Institute had treated more than two thousand patients in the previous six years and could treat even the most severely disabled patients, the ad bragged. "It's nice to know that now there is help," it proclaimed above the red sentence about Dr. Hammesfahr's Nobel Prize nomination, "for his highly successful and revolutionary approach in the treatment of stroke." This Doctor Hammesfahr had been nominated for the 1999 Nobel Prize in Medicine. How do you get nominated for the Nobel Prize? Can anyone nominate? How many nominations are there for each award? Maybe he nominated himself. Does that give him credibility? Or does it make him sound even more bizarre?

There was an 800 number and a web address. I closed the magazine and held it to my chest keeping my finger in the page. What if I closed this magazine and did nothing? No one would know. What kind of responsibility did I have for my father anyway? He lived alone in a retirement hotel. My sister checked in on him every day.

What if the claims were true? What if Dr. Hammesfahr had discovered a revolutionary breakthrough and I didn't let my dad know about it. I held my finger there, thinking for a long time before I opened the magazine again and tore out the advertisement. I glanced over at Steve to see if he had noticed, but he was buried in The Wall Street Journal. I didn't say anything to him. I could keep the ad with me and think about it. I didn't have to act immediately. There was no risk in just keeping the ad.

But it was already too late.

When there is a possibility, when there is a chance, when that word hope starts working on the heart, it creates an open place that is sensitive to the slightest nuance. I didn't want anyone near that place just yet, but it was unmistakably there.

I picked up my book as the plane took off to Chicago and buried my conscious mind in its pre-Camelot melodrama. I put my own unfolding odyssey neatly between the pages of the book to save until I arrived home. But the ad kept slipping out of the pages and peeking into my sight and it was hard to concentrate on the book.

In "The Skystone," Publius and Caius discuss a stone that purportedly fell from the sky. In the fourth century AD, Caius found it difficult to understand how a stone could get into the sky high enough to come down with the amount of force necessary to make so large a crater around it. Publius argued that the stone was not catapulted from the earth, but that it came directly from the stars. To Caius, with his fourth century preconceptions, that was nonsense. The stars were obviously made of light, not stone. Publius, a blacksmith, understood that metal, heated in a forge could glow like light. For him, a stone falling from the sky was possible.

Seventeen hundred years later, with telescopes and probes in outer space, the concept of falling stones seemed easy. Not so easy was the believing that a mute man could talk, or a crippled man could walk, or a mind-muddled man could think, within a few weeks or months of medical treatment.

Could I believe in miracles? From a doctor who advertised in magazines? Who claimed in bright red letters to have been nominated for the 1999 Nobel Prize in medicine and physiology? Could I hope?

2
A Shot in the Dark
September

Without risking my pride, I could look up the web site mentioned in the ad. It was my first task when I got home. The computer took forever to connect to the Internet. I am sure these machines work more slowly when I am in a hurry to remind me that my time sometimes runs fast and sometimes drags along, while theirs is fixed in perfect space. I waited and finally typed in the address. The web site was a medical journal called MedForum.

I found the page with six links and the line, "What's new: Stroke Therapy." Linked to that was a series of articles detailing the procedures used at the Institute. The first thing I noticed was that Dr. Hammesfahr was located on Druid Road East, in Clearwater, Florida. Druid Road? All I needed was a little witchcraft to go along with the red and blue advertisement.

The professional paper covered sixty-seven patients. Eighty-two percent had major improvement, Twelve percent had minor improvement and Six percent showed no improvement. The patients were of all different ages and their strokes had occurred numerous years before they received Dr. Hammesfahr's therapy. No patients worsened.

The majority had improvement by the third office visit. Placebo effect, maybe. But so what? If there was a placebo effect and it worked, then it was a cure. What did I care if it was psychological?

No patients worsened. No patients worsened. It ran like a mantra over and over again. I couldn't hurt my dad. No patients worsened.

In the first few months of my father's slow recovery from his stroke, he often called things by odd names. I wrote them down because in a strange way these misnomers were creative and funny. "Ribbons of numbers" was the stock market streaming along the bottom of the TV screen. "Head bones" was the telephone. "Turn on the spot," meant turn on the light, a reference left over from his many years in community theater. The "over/under score" was his blood pressure. They were almost right. When a brain does not work normally, it finds all kinds of ways to communicate.

The reason I understood how my dad was trying to communicate was because as a child I did not learn to read. I would sit in a circle in the reading group and listen to what the other students read aloud. Then I would try to guess what might come next in the story. I would say that sentence when it was my turn. I created a new plot line for every story in the book. Sometimes mine were better and I was disappointed in the author's version.

Then all of a sudden, in fourth grade, the written word became clear. One day I could not read and the next day I could. I often wondered if all of those phonics lessons Mrs. Snowberger had pounded into my head finally worked, or if synapses in my brain suddenly awoke. When I did read, I read like a fiend. I finished all the reading texts in my one-room schoolhouse in a year. By summer I had graduated to "The Bobbsey Twins" and my own library card. My Aunt Jeanette began to send the "Oz" books. They were just as crazy as my made-up stories. Flowers had personalities and talked, and the Tin Man fell through the center of the earth and popped out on the other side, forever fixing in my mind that the earth was round and had a hole through the center like a wooden bead. Travel to distant lands was obviously very easy.

It was only when I began to teach special education students in a West Side Chicago school that I found out about dyslexia. An "aha!" floated around in my brain as I read the textbooks that described my own childhood experiences of word guessing and avoidance of reading. How could I have been so blind? Why hadn't my education classes in college told me? Right under my nose was the explanation and I had ignored it, or not seen it, or not understood how it related to me, and dismissed it as meaningless.

I wondered why I had not seen anything about the Hammesfahr Neurological Institute until that week. I wondered why there had been no mention of it in the various medical letters to which I subscribed. They told me often enough to beware of saw palmetto and gingko extract. One letter devoted a whole column to the non-existent Vitamin O. Why wasn't there even a paragraph used as filler on Dr. Hammesfahr, when there were endless articles on hopeful experiments with mice?

The ad had suddenly appeared. I was ready to read it. Reading it changed everything. If I had seen it the year before when I was still working every day, when there was no possibility that I could take three weeks off to help my father, I would have closed the magazine, dismissed the ad as quackery and never thought of it again. If I had seen it again I would have thought, oh, there's that flamboyant ad, and turned the page. But the timing was perfect. I had just retired from thirty years of teaching. I had no responsibilities. I was free to do as I pleased. I had lots of time.

There were four preliminary case studies attached to the article. They twisted my heart. The first case was the one quoted in the ad. The woman was the assistant director of a nursing school who had had a stroke during heart surgery two months before. She had profound aphasia. Normal conversation was impossible. She had suffered from migraine headaches and hypertension before the stroke. She now required assistance going up and down stairs and needed a cane. Within forty-eight hours of the beginning of Dr. Hammesfahr's treatment, she could talk and walk and went out boating. She started back to work the next week.

The second case was a fifty-two-year-old house painter. He had had many strokes over the previous five years. He had lost sensation on his left side, his short-term memory was affected, and he developed dyslexia, dizziness, and personality changes. He had constant headaches. He was institutionalized and unable to function in the normal world when he began treatment. In four months, he was well. He began to play his guitar again and he returned to climbing ladders and painting houses.

The third case had immediate improvement to approximately eighty per cent of pre-stroke state. Immediate improvement! It seemed impossible.

The fourth was a sixty-one-year-old neurologist who had peer-reviewed Dr. Hammesfahr's article about the work being done on strokes at the Hammesfahr Neurological Institute. The neurologist reported to the Institute within eleven hours of his stroke. He had trouble speaking, or aphasia, word substitution, mild dyslexia, mental confusion, and agraphia, the inability to write. He was treated and went back to work the next day. The minute he forgot to take his medications however, the symptoms returned. Here was another affirmation, this one by a fellow physician.

I looked up Dr. Hammesfahr's resume with the American Medical Association. It stated that he was an honor student graduate of Northwestern University's Medical School in neurology and that he had done his residency at the College of Virginia. Those were very reputable schools. This man was a real doctor, not some quack. That was enough for me.

My heart began to pound. I decided to talk it over with Steve, my always-cautious companion.

"It sounds interesting," he said. "Why don't you ask your doctor about the treatment? Maybe she will know something about it."

"Do you think I should tell my father?"

"Yes. He's a grown man. Let him decide." Steve returned to his stock market calculations.

If I called my father and told him what I'd found, I knew that with that glimmer of hope he would make a snap decision. He was not afraid of change. I thought he would try anything in order to get rid of the constant pain in his tensed right arm and leg. I had no perfect choices. If I didn't tell him, I would feel guilty because I might have helped him. If I did tell him, and the treatment didn't work, it would be my fault. I weighed the consequences. I tried to make a decision. I decided not to decide just yet.

I called the Hammesfahr Neurological Institute to ask if they had any information about the treatment. Someone answered on the first ring.

"Hammesfahr Neurological Institute. This is Debbie. May I help you?"

I had a real person on the line when I had expected an answering machine. She was there. I was nervous.

"Do you, uh, treat strokes?" I flubbed my first line.

"Yes we do. Can I help you?"

"My father had a stroke eight years ago," I began. "Can you help him?"

"Absolutely!" she said. There was no equivocation. There was unbridled enthusiasm in this voice. "It doesn't matter when he had the stroke."

"He also had some bleeding in the brain. Doctors drilled holes in his head to alleviate it. Does that make a difference?"

REVERSING THE RAVAGES OF STROKE   27

"Not at all. How old is your father?"

"Does that matter?"

"No, I just want to take down some information about him."

"He's eighty-two. He doesn't have anything else the matter with him except he has prostate cancer. He takes hormones for that."

"No problem. The initial treatment using standard therapy will take three weeks." She asked me a few more questions. "I can send you some information about the Institute and Dr. Hammesfahr. There's also a video tape of Dr. Hammesfahr in the information package that explains the treatment," she said. "I'll put it in the mail today." She took my address. "Where did you hear about this Institute?"

"I saw it in an airline magazine ad."

"A lot of people see it there. Have you seen the MedForum web site?

"Yes, that's why I called."

"I'll send you all the information today. Your father may need to have tests run with his general practitioner before he comes here. And we will need his medical records, especially the ones regarding the stroke. His release papers from the hospital should have it all. This information will all be in the package I'm sending you."

"Thank you," I said. Thank you, thank you, thank you, I thought as we hung up. I loved the idea of getting more information. As a teacher, I was confident only when I knew everything there was to know about a subject. No matter what crazy questions the students came up with, I could say, "I don't know" only so many times and I had better show up the next day with the answer. I felt more powerful now that I knew there was more information I would soon possess.

I called my sister, Lia, Dad's primary caregiver, and told her about the therapy.

"Well," she said, after I had explained everything. She sounded tired. "I'll look it up on the web. Call me when you find out more from their office."

But she really meant leave me alone. It was a short conversation without much enthusiasm. It made me want to think a bit more before going ahead.

3
New Ideas
Later September

The next day I had an appointment with my doctor. It was for a general check-up, so I had no personal worries, just worries about Dad. After the examination, when I had my clothes on again, I told the doctor about the possibility of treatment for him.

"My father had a stroke in a small town." I said. "I worry about older doctors in small towns. I am afraid they might not know the latest techniques or have the most up-to-date information. I've worked with teachers to try to get them to change, and I know that many teachers like to stick with techniques they learned in school. If doctors are anything like those teachers, I don't have a great deal of faith in them."

"I understand exactly where you are coming from," she replied. "My dad had diabetes. I finally said, 'Look, Dad, I'm a doctor now. Let me see your charts and let me tell you what you should do.' I ordered a few more tests and found that he had an artery about ready to pop. If I hadn't taken the trouble, it might have. The average GP just doesn't have time to check everything."

My doctor is young with long blonde hair. She doesn't look like a doctor, and she wasn't talking like one either. I'd never had a doctor tell me about personal experiences before, not in my entire life.

"I have studies I got off of the web," I said, "about a stroke treatment that is being used at the Hammesfahr Neurological Institute in Clearwater, Florida. The doctor was trained at Northwestern University Medical School. I am trying to decide whether to take my father down to try this treatment. They say that eighty-two percent of the patients have major improvement. Can that be true? Am I being taken in by something? Would you look at this material and give me your advice?"

She sat down and began reading the summary at the beginning of one of the articles. I waited.

She flipped through the pages, skimming them quickly. It seemed like a long time before she looked up.

"Medically, I don't see anything in this treatment that could hurt him," she began. "Have you told your father about it?"

"No, I wanted to wait until I was sure that it was not a scam. I don't want to raise his hopes if there is nothing to it."

"There are doctors in this world who discover things that work. He could be one of them. Many things have been learned that way, or through serendipity. Medicine is an art, as well as a science. In medicine, we are still in the stages of bloodletting and leeches. Do you know how we treat cancer? We poison the patient with radiation and chemicals. Medical treatment in the next twenty years will be entirely different from now. Mapping the human gnomes and advances in studying the genes will revolutionize this profession.

"If your father wants to do this, I recommend that you go ahead. If he has hope, even a little hope, for a little while, it is important. You can't hurt him. Maybe it will make him better." She handed the papers back to me.

Frankly, I was astounded. I could not believe that a doctor would be so open to new ideas. I hadn't known doctors except the patronizing ones, or the too-busy kind. Mine was a real exception. She talked to me as though I was an intelligent human being who could understand what she was saying. As though I would heed her advice, along with the other things that I was considering about this treatment, weigh the evidence, and make a decision. What a difference that made! I felt so much better that I went home filled with expectation.

My dad, who was a retired psychologist and college professor, had new ideas and many disagreements with universities over his choices. He used an unpopular direct psychotherapy to counsel students at a time when the Carl Rogers style of indirect counseling was in vogue. Dad understood it, but didn't agree with it. He wanted the students he worked with to confront their problems, even if they were sexual ones. Now the world understands the more direct style of Dr. Phil and other therapists. Talking about sex is no longer forbidden but it was not acceptable in the 1950s when students he was counseling brought up the subject. Both my dad and I understood what a "new idea" meant and the ramifications that it had for career and family. For a while there, we moved to a new university every year.

Dad came to the conclusion that people learn and grow, not in spite of setbacks, but because of them. If we shunned setbacks we stopped learning. He thought that we should embrace them as a step towards new knowledge. As Thomas Edison once said, "I have not failed. I've just found 10,000 ways that won't work."

That night, I stayed awake reading until midnight and even then I couldn't fall asleep. I needed to consult my sister, Lia, and I was concerned about her reaction. Her specter loomed over my bed. Irrational fear and worry washed over me again. My father could be hurt or even die because of this treatment. I would be the cause. I ran through all of the moments in my head. Why had I gotten myself into this? Well, I could take the easiest way out. I could retreat. I didn't need to call Lia. I didn't need to call the Institute for an appointment. I didn't have to do anything at all.

My last thought as I drifted toward sleep was about my friend Maureen, who has an inner voice that talks to her and tells her to do the craziest things.

When she was going into the hospital for the exploratory surgery on her lung, she decided that she wanted to see a hypnotist before the operation. I could hear her expressive voice begin the story.

"I was driving back to Riverside from school and a little voice said to me (here she shifted into a high pitched squeak), 'Why don't you go down North Avenue to Harlem and take Harlem home?'

"That's ridiculous," her conscious mind replied. "No one ever goes that way. I've never gone that way." Maureen shook her head. But she turned down North Avenue.

Her inner voice said, "You are going to pass a park. Watch."

Maureen drove on by the park, but the voice said, "Turn here."

"That's enough," her conscious mind responded. "It's an Old Navy store. There is no hypnotist in an Old Navy Store." She remembered that the only night she had available before surgery was Thursday, and then not until late.

She arrived home and opened the phone book. There was only one number for a hypnotist in Riverside. The number contained her birth date. Another coincidence. A man answered the phone rather brusquely.

"Do you hypnotize people?" Maureen asked. "I am going to have surgery."

"Oh," he relaxed and sounded much friendlier. "That's what I do. Most of the time I work with patients at Oak Park Hospital."

"Do you have a private practice?"

"Yes, but I work only on Thursday nights and I don't have an open appointment until late."

"Perfect," Maureen said. "Where are you located?"

"Behind the Old Navy Store on Harlem Avenue. Drive into the parking lot because you can't see the sign for the office from the street."

Those kinds of things were always happening to Maureen. Her inner voices were always giving her messages. My inner voices never talked to me, or maybe they had but I never listened. When Maureen followed through with these intuitive suggestions, she invariably came up with a solution to her latest knotty problem. I surely could've used that kind of intuition. I needed an inner voice or at least a sign. I wished for a sign.

My transcendental meditation teacher said that there are hundreds of signs each day. We simply don't notice them. I vowed that I would be aware and waiting the next day. With that thought firmly planted in my dream-ready mind, I finally fell asleep.

4
A New Light
The Next Day

I had no intuitive dreams. Figures.

I had to take my four-year-old grandson to pre-school before the nine o'clock deadline. The previous week when he'd slept over, I'd been twelve minutes late and had to pay a six dollar fine. I wasn't going to get caught like that again. It was a thirty-minute bike ride to his pre-school, but it was a lovely ride through Lincoln Park and along the lakefront bike path. My grandson kept pointing out sailboats and dogs and airplanes in the early morning air. When we got to school, he greeted everyone by name. His classmates greeted me with "Hi, Miss Grandma." My worries from the previous night, about subjecting my father to an unknown therapy, were cleansed away by the night wizards, the morning sunlight and the enthusiastic children. Each day was wondrous for them. They lived each moment to its fullest. They did not think about tomorrow.

On the way home, I stopped to buy tomatoes and basil at the organic farmer's market in the Chicago Historical Society parking lot. I put them in my basket and pedaled over to the beach bike path. There wasn't a cloud in the sky. It was so pure blue that the haze of smog that sometimes hangs near the lake's horizon had disappeared. I stopped my bike and got off in a spot where nothing was visible except the water and the horizon.

I'd been learning to paint with watercolors, bringing my paints to the lakefront and working on water and skies. I had glorious green skies, yellow and pink skies, purple skies and gray skies, but was not nearly as successful with water. Somehow my water kept coming out looking solid blue, instead of having waves and glints. So I stopped to look carefully at the water in hope of getting some hint as to how to paint it.

Suddenly, I noticed that the sun was making the water shine in a broad V-shaped path that came right to me. Around it, the water on either side was deep blue. The path of golden sunlight was so strong it looked as though I could walk on it. It was my own yellow brick road. Then I realized. It's a sign. It's a big enough sign that even I can recognize it.

Right out there in the middle of the park, I did the yoga movements for Sun Salutation and filled my body with energy. Light and birds always made me think of my mother's spirit, of how good it felt when my mother touched my face or stroked my cheek. When she died, I thought her energy faded into the light, and would be reflected back in a thousand fragmented glints. Like the pictures of Aten, the Egyptian sun god, her long light arms could reach out and embrace me. Although I don't know whether I believe in specific angels watching over me, I thanked her for the sign, anyway.

I could never have taken away the hope that this trip and this treatment would give my father. I had dared to hope and I had infected myself with longing for him to be whole again. We would take an odyssey together. Like all journeys, the traveling would be as important as the destination.

I could not wait to call my dad to see if he would be willing to embark upon this quest. Of course, he could say no. It could be beyond his wildest possibilities. He could be too afraid to change. Maybe he was satisfied where he was and as he was. Maybe it would be too much effort for him. But I was convinced. I could offer him this possibility. If he did not wish to do it, so be it.

I called him. My heart was in my throat and I was afraid that I would not be able to talk. What if I was over-confident? What if I was wrong? Doubts lingered.

5
I Would Rather Die
Same Day

The phone rang several times before my father picked it up. I could hear CNBC on the television in the background. He left the TV on all the time, watching the ribbons of stock market numbers go by, listening to the analysis of the financial talking heads, and more often than not, dozing.

"Hi, Dad," I began. "Good day in the market?"

"Robin, let me turn this squawk box off so I can hear you." Background noise severely interfered with his hearing. I heard him fumble for the remote.

"Dag-blasted thing fell into my chair." He had the cord pinned to his recliner chair so that it wouldn't fall to the floor. If it did, it would be difficult for him to pick it up. "My girl is here," he continued in his old-fashioned way. "She's cleaning up." The woman washed his clothes, stripped his bed, cleaned his bathroom, vacuumed, and dusted. She also washed out his coffee cups and drinking glasses. These were all things he could not do, and the reasons why my sister had insisted that he leave his ranch-style home in western Illinois, and move to Rock Island, to The Fort Armstrong, a retirement hotel near her.

"I hurt, Robin. The muscles inside my back are jumping on the right side, if you know what I mean by jumping. It's what happens when you double up a fist hard and hold it. Soon all the muscles start jumping. The pain comes out of my back all the way into my arm." I could hear him take a deep breath.

"My hand clamped shut on me in the middle of the night last night. I've spent the morning trying to get it pried open with my other hand. The pain goes from my fingers, up my elbow and makes a circular curve in my upper arm. And the market is terrible," Dad complained.

"I'm sorry Dad," I said knowing that I could do little to help him. "Have you taken your Ibuprofen?"

"Yes. It does nothing against the pain."

"I have a proposition that may cheer you up," I said.

"I could use some cheering up. This place is like a funeral home. Two people got carted off yesterday."

"Did you know them?"

"No, but one guy keeled over into his mashed potatoes at lunch time."

"Is he okay?"

"No, he's dead. The other one got hauled out while he was playing bridge."

"You do need this cheering up, Dad."

"I sure do. I feel like I don't have a life of my own. I get pushed around and I do what I'm told. Everybody else makes decisions for me. I used to look out of my house at the swimming pool going to rack and ruin. Nobody took care of it like I did. When I had to sell the house I didn't have any say in it. I figured, 'What the heck I'd just come to this place where they took care of old people and stay here until I died. I feel powerless." His voice was stoic and emotionless.

"Oh, Dad." I didn't know what to say because what he said happened was true, but he couldn't stay at home alone.

He and Lia had looked at several other places before choosing the Fort Armstrong. At the first one, the building itself looked unfriendly. It was a new building where everything was polished brick. It looked like a perfect setup. It had modern furniture and modern everything else, but it didn't have any of the warmth Dad wanted. The Fort Armstrong was a little homier, at least.

"You kids think I'm a nuisance," Dad went on. "It is hard to describe how I feel. My whole life is tearing apart. One shred of it goes in one direction and another shred of it goes in another direction."

"Dad, don't you have friends there? Everybody likes you."

"It's like when I started in the Air Force in WW II. Everyone else was just like you. They were soldiers stuck on a base in Florida and they couldn't do anything about it. They suddenly were thrown into a world of strangers and told to make friends. I know if I don't do that here, I'll just sit here and die."

"You make my heart ache," I said.

"This is how I feel, not what is actually happening. I know this is not a dumping ground for me. It's going to be up to me to make the best of it that I can. It's just this pain in my leg is killing me. My hip feels like the bone joint is out of place and it hurts when I walk. The pain goes clear down the side of my leg and my foot. I feel like my foot is constantly being charged with electricity and it gives me shocks every time I take a step." He spoke haltingly, searching for words.

"I know something that might help. Let me tell you my news. I found a doctor who is treating stroke victims with a great deal of success. I don't know if he can help you, but there is a possibility that he can."

"Help me with what?"

"He has had some success with paralysis, aphasia, improving walking, all the problems you have."

"What do you mean 'some success'?"

"I mean eighty-two percent of his patients had major improvement, eleven percent had some improvement and the rest had no improvement."

"I'll go. Where is he?"

"Clearwater, Florida."

"I could get there," he said almost to himself. I knew that he was wondering how he could take care of himself if he did go. "Is this a hospital?"

"No, Dad, it's a doctor's clinic. I would go with you for the three weeks they say it takes to set up your medicines. But before you commit to this, you need to listen to the downside. It is possible that you could have another stroke and get worse.

"I could have another stroke right here, at any time. I want to go. I'd do anything to get rid of this constant pain."

"It is possible that you will undergo the treatment and not get any better. Maybe there will be something about your situation that will keep them from taking you at all."

"I would rather die than continue like this."

My heart jumped a beat at that fearsome thought.

There was a silence as I struggled for words to respond to the thought of my father's death or worse, suicide. I'd read all the statistics about old people and gunshot deaths. Dad's grandfather had committed suicide. I remembered Hemingway.

"I'll go with you. We can take a Florida vacation together. It will be fun."

"Oh, you don't have to do that," he said, ever confident.

"I want to do it. We can get a motel room with a swimming pool and go to the Institute every day. We'll have a great time, even if nothing changes in your condition."

"Will you set it up?"

"I'll send you all the case studies I got off of the web. Get someone to read them aloud to you. I'll call the Institute."

"I have a doctor's appointment in two days," Dad said. I could talk to him about this therapy."

"I'll send him the case studies I have this afternoon. Then he can look at them before he sees you."

"This has cheered me up enormously. I was down in a hole and now I can see light at the top. Thank you, Robin."

"Nothing to it, Dad. I love you."

"I love you, too." We hung up.

I sent the information from the Lifeline Journal at MedForum web page to dad's new doctor via overnight express mail. I included a letter requesting that dad's medical records be given to him at his next office visit. It cost me twenty-three dollars, but I figured if I could give the doctor a few days to look at the studies, it would be well worth it.

When Dad broached the idea of the Hammesfahr Neurological Institute to his doctor a few days later, the doctor said, "You don't want to do that. It's a waste of your time and your money." The twenty-three dollar envelope lay unopened on the desk right beside Dad's chair. "Let my receptionist make an appointment with a neurologist here."

"I left the office disgusted," Dad told me on the phone that night. "The doctor didn't want to hear any of it. And he treated me as though I were a child, and a not too bright child, at that. I don't like that man."

Needless to say, since the doctor had not read my letter, he did not give my father a copy of his medical records. It didn't sound as though we were going to get the cooperation we needed from him.

It was going to be difficult to gather all of Dad's medical information without his doctor's assistance. I had to start working with my sister right away, and I was worried about how she was going to react to this new, more urgent, demand. If she did not approve of this treatment it would be difficult for Dad and me to proceed. She was the one who would have to administer the medicines and keep track of his progress. I wanted her to be a part of the therapy. She was my next call.

6
Dissent
The Last Week of September

I called Lia to tell her what we would need to take to the Institute. Dad's current doctor should send us (fat chance) his latest tests, blood work and the hospital discharge papers from his stroke. She responded in monosyllables.

My sister had spent three years caring for our mother, as stroke after stroke left her more and more debilitated. Once a vivacious teacher and learner, mother had deteriorated to her final non-walking, non-talking, one-armed state, as Lia watched her fail, watched the doctors do nothing. There was nothing they knew to do. There was nothing they could do.

Each week there was another series of setbacks. If there was a day when mother felt well, it was followed by two days when she felt worse.

My sister was there on the day Mother's tooth fell out. My mother had been a good-looking woman. She'd prided herself on her unique style and flirtatious smile. When she asked for a mirror my sister cringed, but brought it to her anticipating the anguish in mother's face when she looked into the mirror saw the bleak reflection of her once beautiful face, now without a front tooth.

My sister was there on the day mother began having seizures, and waited with her until the ambulance came. Mother was terrified of being tied down ever since she'd had eye operations as an eight-year-old child. In that primitive time, 1926, the doctors scraped the growths off her eyes using ether on one day and no ether, but simply restraints to tie her down the next day. She never recovered emotionally. She clutched at my sister as the medics put her in restraints and loaded her into the ambulance, her eyes pleading for Lia to prevent this atrocity from happening. My sister was helpless

I was there giving Lia a bit of respite the weekend when Mother, suddenly, could no longer swallow. She was weak and dehydrated when she got up from her afternoon nap, and could not get her pills or even water down her throat. She could not eat. Dad and I were calm and terrified at the same time. Even with her "do not resuscitate" and "no extraordinary means" requests, even though we thought we knew that she wanted to die, we put her into the hospital that weekend and authorized an IV of fluids to keep her hydrated. We let them feed her with a tube down her throat. We let them operate on her gall bladder. We let her live in abject agony. It was more comfortable for us.

Like many people, we went along with what the doctor said to do. We knew what she was doing when she ripped the IVs out of her arm over and over again. We saw in her eyes the pleading to let her die.

I could not do it. Nor could my sister or my father.

Day after day she begged us to end everything. For nine long weeks in the hospital, having withered to sixty-five pounds and undergone an emergency gall bladder operation, she willed herself dead. Lia watched her go. My mother, my sister, my father, and I were all helpless and angry.

I knew my sister had gut-wrenching feelings of guilt because she had not been able to act when mother was pleading for her to end her life. Although it had been three years earlier, Lia still had nightmares every few nights. Once she told me, "I dream that I'll be in the same position as Mother, that I will be the one not able to talk or walk. The horror will be me, like Mother, not ever getting better. I awake in intense fear. I have to get out of bed and do something else in the middle of the night to rid myself of these terrors."

I knew all of that. I didn't like to think about it. But I knew it. Still, I called to ask for her help.

"I don't want anything to do with your plan," Lia said in a monotone. "I have seen enough doctors and enough hospitals and enough death. If you want to do it, go ahead, but leave me out of it."

"I need your help." There was along pause at the end of the line. I listened to her silent plea to leave her alone. "I need all his medical records from the stroke," I said, trying to get her to work with me. There was another long pause.

"What if he has another stroke? I don't want to be pushing a wheel chair around." I could picture her stoic face, set hard, her hand running through her short brown hair, her blue eyes that looked just like Dad's tense and worried.

"What if he gets better?" I countered. "What if he can walk well again? What if the pain stops?" She was again, silent. I waited. "Even if he gets no better, isn't it worth trying? Would you rather do nothing?"

"He could die." I finally heard softly from my sister. There was another long pause.

"No patient worsened in this treatment." I repeated my mantra to her. But I knew that she was too tied to her personal pain to hear me.

"Look, Dad wants to do it. If he wants to do it, he should do it," she said in the same tired voice. I heard her glasses click on the kitchen countertop. I knew just where she was standing, in front of the refrigerator, looking over the counter, out the big picture window in the den.

Beyond that window lay the carefully planted front yard she had worked on since Mother's death. She had transplanted many of the wildflowers that Mother had collected over the years from the farms of friends and neighbors. She had jack-in-the-pulpit, trillium, false Solomon seal, Virginia blue bells, and old-fashioned yellow and brown iris. They did not die. They grew and prospered. She could not control Mom's illness, but she could control that garden.

"Did you see the information I sent about the treatment?" There was only breathing at the end of the line.

"Are you all right?" I heard her exhale a big puff of tension.

"I have a cold. I have had it all week. I don't care what you do. Don't call me about this any more."

"All right," I said. There was a click on the end of the line and Lia was gone. I listened to the empty space go on and on.

Once I took a transcendental meditation class. The guru had names for all of the meditations he taught us. Things like "Go With the Flow" and "Send Out Love." One that I particularly liked was the "Cosmic Sigh." You used it in a situation that seemed impossible, one that was going to cause a lot of problems and you had no power to change. There was nothing to do but continue on the path you had begun, even if it led to disaster. In this frustrating position a huge sigh helped. I used the Cosmic Sigh once. Then I used it again.

My sister had just said that she would not help me. I could do nothing about that. I called my two brothers, one older and one younger, and told them about the Institute. The younger one said, "Go for it." They both expressed hope that it would work, but neither of them was much interested in researching the medical procedure or helping, other than to offer moral support. They were far away in Milwaukee and Dallas, and both had their own families and their own jobs.

Their busy lives filled their time and took all of their energy, just as mine had the year before.

I was the only one not working. I had the time to take Dad to Clearwater and stay with him for the three-week treatment. After everything my sister had done for our mother, it was my turn. I whined to myself, "Yeah, but I helped her when she took care of mother. She could at least be supportive of me." I still didn't want the whole responsibility for this venture. There were too many unanswered questions and chances. If I was wrong....

I called my father and told him what had happened. "Lia was so apathetic. And disinterested." I ranted. "And negative."

"I don't want you two to fight." Dad spoke quietly. I suddenly realized how uncomfortable he was on the other end of the line. "I'm going to do what I want to do and I want to go to Clearwater. If you'll take me, that is."

"Of course I'll take you."

"Good. Just leave your sister alone."

"Did she say anything to you about not wanting you to go?"

"Her husband gave me this article. The title is "Magnetic Resonance Imaging-Ischemia." Each of the words he struggled through. "Patho-phys-iol-ogy. Robin, I can't read this."

I used another Cosmic Sigh. "Send it to me in the mail. Why is Lia mad at me? We are always on the same side."

"Robin, you can go over this and go over this, but it is not going to change anything."

"I'll stop. I promise." I am being petty and vindictive, I thought. I'd better shut my mouth. "I'm going to hang up, Dad. I can't talk now or I'll just go on and on and sound terrible. I love you."

"I love you, too."

A soft end to hard talk.

I went into the office to tell Steve about it. Talking to him always helped. It must be something about his engineering background that makes him think so logically and unemotionally.

"Your father wants to go. He supports you. You don't need anyone else," was his advice.

Still, I hated the idea of proceeding without Lia's cooperation. I don't like acting alone. My whole adult life I was a schoolteacher and involved with committee after committee. Committees run schools. Now I had made this decision alone and I didn't want to do it alone. I was miserable.

Lists always make me feel as though I am in control, so I listed the reasons why I shouldn't take Dad to the Institute:

If the treatment failed, everyone would blame me.

If nothing happened, they would laugh at me behind my back.

Or criticize me for spending their inheritance.

This treatment could actually harm him.

The reasons why I shouldn't do it were all weak and negative. I listed the reasons why I should do it:

I was a big girl. I could take the blame if I was wrong.

I have been laughed at before. I didn't wither away.

Dad was spending his own money. He earned it. What better way to spend it than on his health?

The Institute said that no patient worsened.

The reasons why I should do it were positive and courageous.

I had yet to meet Dr. Hammesfahr and did not yet know the personal trauma that inextricably moved him through life towards his amazing discovery. I was still struggling with the pros and cons.

7
Action
The Next Day

I called the Institute. Once again, Debbie answered the phone. "This is Robin Robinson. I want to make an appointment for my father, Dr. Edward W. Robinson. How soon can we get one?" There was a short pause.

"We have time available on the third of October and on the ninth of October."

I made the appointment for the third of October, three weeks away.

"You are aware that his procedure currently is not covered by Medicare." Debbie said. "There is a $5,000 charge, payable when you arrive at the Institute."

"Why doesn't Medicare cover it?" I asked.

"They did until a few months ago. They wanted to investigate the therapy so they put a hold on payments to the Institute until they were finished. We are in the process of appealing the decision." (Medicare has since reinstated payment.)

"We still want the appointment," I said. But the rejection of Dad's insurance was another entry on my list of doubts.

"There is information in the materials I am sending about local motels that give our patients a discount. Please send in the medical information in the packet as soon as you can. See you in October."

When I got the package, I pulled out the page with a list of ten motels.

I decided to call the non-chain hotels first, with the thought they might have a special set-up that would work for Dad and me. The Aloha Motel was a friendly sounding name. I dialed.

"We have a set of two rooms at the back of the motel next to the canal. They are away from the street noise and might suit you and your father. They were originally designed for the owner's two children. There is a kitchen between the two living rooms and two separate bedrooms and bathrooms." It sounded ideal.

"How much are they?"

"This is off season so I can let you have them for $350 a week. Are you coming on vacation?"

"No, my Dad is going to the Hammesfahr Neurological Institute for three weeks. We'll need the rooms for October 2nd through October 23rd. Are you close to the Institute?"

"About two miles. We've had patients from that place before. They all seem to get better before they leave."

"Really," I responded. "That is heartening news." This was important! It was an unbiased observation by a stranger.

"Are you a computer person? If so, pull up our web site, fill out the registration, and e-mail it to us."

On the web site there was a greeting from Bud and Monica, the owners, and a description of the place. It was "friendly, family-oriented, very clean, spacious, had wall-to-wall carpeting, air conditioning, and a cable-connected TV." There were pictures of a small swimming pool and a fishing pier that overlooked Clearwater Bay. It looked fine.

My adrenaline was on high as I called Dad to let him know the information from the Institute was on its way. I had to dial three times in order to get the number right, a little dyslexic kickback.

"Hey, Dad, what are you up to?" I asked.

"About five-foot-ten," he shot back the punch line for the joke he had been using for at least fifty years. "And you?"

He must be feeling good today. So often he was sad.

"Up to your shoulder," I teased. "I made an appointment with Dr. Hammesfahr and booked the flights and motel. We have an appointment in three weeks, Dad."

"Why not sooner?" he asked.

"That's the first one I could get. It's going to cost $5,000 for the three weeks of therapy. I guess that is not a lot as far as doctors go, but they also said that Medicare would not cover it. You have to be prepared to actually pay for it. Do you still want to go if it's that expensive?"

"Of course I still want to go. I've got enough money. I can cover it." My father grew up during the depression and was careful about his money. While I was growing up in the 50's we had numerous money-raising projects to supplement his teaching income. We raised baby chicks, pure-breed collies and had an ill-fated experience with rabbits which failed when we couldn't soften the rabbit hides. Dad suggested that mother chew them, but she refused.

"Robin, I am in such pain that I cry myself to sleep at night. I will try almost anything to stop my misery. Right now I wish I could sleep all the time. It is the only time I am not in pain."

"Then get your suitcase out and pack all your shorts. We're going to Florida."

"I've got a letter from my doctor here." I could hear him unfold the pages.

"What did it say?"

"He is closing his practice and going to work for a corporation."

"That explains it! No wonder he wasn't interested in getting involved with you."

I hung up the phone. Taking action was very exhilarating. We'd made the commitment. The appointment was barely three weeks away. We had a lot to do.

My sister called that night. I didn't start the conversation. I waited until I heard what she had to say. "I have Dad's medical records from Dr. Ball. They're from his last time in surgery, when he had the hernia. I can't get the records from his GP. The office is just not cooperative."

Lia had done what she said she was not going to do. She had an incredible amount of strength.

"Did Dad tell you about the letter from his doctor?" she continued.

"Yes. No wonder the doctor wasn't cooperative. Do you think you could get his hospital release records after his stroke?" I asked. "I tried County Hospital and they wouldn't send them. They said it was too long ago."

"I don't know," Lia said.

"Well, send whatever you get along with Dad when he comes to me in Chicago. I'll make copies of everything before we go to Clearwater."

8
Adventure Travel
Three Weeks Later

Three weeks later, dad arrived in Chicago after a bizarre set of events. My sister took him to the Greyhound Bus Station, after first calling Greyhound to ascertain what time the bus to Chicago would leave Rock Island, but when they arrived at the station, there was no bus.

"There isn't going to be one, either," the lone attendant informed them with a Midwestern twang. "Not today, anyway."

Lia called Greyhound's main number again. They reassured her that there was going to be a bus. Finally, when it became obvious that there was no bus, the attendant suggested that they call Act II Limousine Company Dad arrived at my house in style, if a little later and a little more expensively than he'd planned. He struggled up the back stairs one by one to my second floor apartment, placing his left foot on a step and then putting his right foot on a step beside it before proceeding to the next step. He stopped on each landing to catch his breath. Steve followed behind him with the luggage, in case he fell backwards.

The first thing I did was pull out Dad's medical files from his suitcase to make copies for Dr. Hammesfahr. The records from his last surgery with Dr. Ball were there and so were the County Hospital records of his stroke from eight years ago.

"How did Lia get these hospital records?" I asked Dad.

"I'm not going to tell you. You ask her how she got them. She's going to enjoy telling you, and I am not going to ruin that conversation."

The next day, Steve drove us to Midway Airport. Dad usually used a cane, but in airports he had to walk long distances and people could knock against him and topple him over, so he always got a wheelchair. It came with an attendant who not only pushed the chair, but also arranged for our luggage to be checked.

While the rest of the passengers stood in a long line to get their seating assignments, we checked in quickly at the handicapped counter. Traveling with a handicapped person was turning out to be a wonderful airport experience. Our plane was due to take off in an hour. Dad hobbled off to the men's room near the gate.

Before Dad got back, the loud speaker blared, "Flight ATA 517 has changed boarding gates. It will now leave from Gate B-12." So much for my gloating. Now I had to figure out how to balance the pull-bag with all of Dad's medical records, carry my big purse, and push the wheelchair. Suddenly, traveling with a handicapped person didn't seem like so much fun.

"We're off on the road to Morocco," Dad quipped as we maneuvered back out to the main concourse. The B gates were in a wing about three blocks away. We dodged fast moving passengers with suitcases, and had to stop on more than one occasion to avoid a collision with an unobservant traveler. We went through the x-ray with assistance from one of the airline workers, and faced the long corridor. Gate B-12 was at the very end.

"I'd whistle a merry tune, but I can't whistle anymore," Dad said. He used to sing these songs with a trained voice that rattled the windows. After the stroke, his voice was weak and scratchy and he stopped singing. "That is a terrible thing, to have lost your whistle. Now you can't even whistle while I work," I huffed as I pushed my heavy load. "I like the part about your working. I never would have made it over here in time for the plane. Thanks for the push."

We boarded the plane first, another little perk for a passenger in a wheelchair.

I flipped through the magazine in the pocket in front of me. There was no heart-stopping advertisement that said "Help for Stroke Victims," just the usual luggage and briefcase ads aimed at business travelers. When I thought about it, I was amazed that I'd even seen the ad that got Dad and me to our airplane seats.

I have always felt as though I was in a state of inaction. That I was stuck in one place and nothing would ever change. I remember as a teenager I thought I would never grow up and get to live like Nick and Nora Charles did on TV. I would never go out with a man in a tuxedo or wear a long gown or drink a martini. I longed to attend an exciting party or historical ball. But I was stuck in a small town in Nebraska, where the biggest event was the summer fair and the biggest prize was for apple preserves or embroidery. I thought that I was trapped there forever. I wasn't.

I wondered if there was a single moment when Dad realized that he was trapped in his body and that he would never get better. I wondered at what moment he might have lost all hope of recovery. Important changes in life occurred in a split second and made the difference between being lonely or in love, bored or fascinated, without purpose or beginning a quest? Was there a point upon which each life balanced or a star that determined when it was time to change? Was life measured in sections, some holding only teaspoons and some holding whole cups? Was there a bigger purpose to our trip? Would it change our lives?

I looked over at Dad, who was already asleep, his handsome face relaxed and free from pain. We went speeding through the sky above the clouds in a time capsule, waiting for change.

Another wheelchair met us at the Tampa airport. I parked Dad next to our luggage while I went to get the rental car. The air smelled damp. My dry nose began to recover immediately.

The Aloha Motel was located on the Clearwater Harbor side of the road, between the Clearwater Bay and Stevenson Creek. Our rooms were at the back of the two-building compound, bordering a canal where birds, fish, and boats edged slowly towards the Gulf. The views were spectacular from both the pool and the fishing pier and boat dock. Tall water birds were feeding in the shallows - herons, egrets, and ibis, along with the terns and gulls. What a fortuitous choice.

Out my window, a gray pelican with a white head and little beady eyes sat hunched down on a pier post. It took off and glided just inches above the water. It landed with a huge splash, tail in the air and beak under water, wings still spread to balance the underwater struggle with a fish. The bird bounced three or four times, then pulled itself right side up and enjoyed its culinary conquest. After a few minutes, it took off with several preliminary flaps of huge bent wings, pushing its webbed feet against the water and dragging its spread tail feathers for three or four wing beats. It rose into the air, did a sharp right turn and dove again. It ate. It dove. It ate. Over and over.

Repetitive actions like taking a shower, getting himself dressed, brushing his teeth, and feeding himself were struggles for Dad. Sometimes, he didn't think it was worth the effort to do them, so his body or his breath smelled bad.

He'd lost his sense of smell with the stroke and that hadn't helped.

We settled into the motel rooms. I unpacked and put our things in drawers. "Do you want to go shopping?" I suggested. "We could get some stuff for dinner and breakfast."

"No, they may not take me tomorrow. If I have to go home, we'd just waste the things we bought."

"Why do you think that they won't take you?"

"There are those holes the doctors drilled in my head. Or my blood pressure could be too low. Who knows?"

I knew that he meant the holes that the doctors had drilled through his skull to relieve the pressure from bleeding inside of his head. This had occurred about a year after his stroke. "They're going to take you," I assured him, although I had no more knowledge on the subject than he did.

"Let's go out to dinner. We didn't have lunch today. I'm hungry."

"They didn't feed us, but it was a cheap flight," I countered. "I'll go ask the owner of the motel for a restaurant recommendation."

The sunset over the Gulf of Mexico lit the sky with gold and pink and lavender as we drove up the road to Dunedin to a lovely waterfront restaurant called 'bon appetit.' We decided to eat fish sandwiches outside on the dock with the breeze and the remnants of the sunset and the pelicans swooping for their dinner just yards away. Since the stroke Dad had lost his sense of taste. He didn't care much what he ate, but he always tried to order food that he could eat with one hand and did not need to be cut. A knife and fork required that both hands work. His right hand stayed clutched next to his chest. A sandwich and French fries he could handle without being embarrassed by his crippled arm. He couldn't feel the right side of his face and he frequently dribbled from that side of his mouth so he didn't want to eat anything messy. Being able to feed himself in a restaurant made him feel that he had some control over his own life.

Back at the motel, I opened the windows before we went to bed, letting in the night air and the sound of water lapping against the edge of the canal. The palm fronds rustled in the wind like hovering angels' wings.

I prayed.

9
Clear Sailing in Clearwater
Tuesday, October 3
Day One

That first day it was difficult to wait for our two o'clock appointment at the Institute. Before breakfast, I had to take Dad's blood pressure and pulse. The readings were low. I wrote them on the sheet the Institute had provided in the information packet. We drove down quiet streets looking for a coffee shop and ended up on the other side of town at the Tin Can Restaurant.

Colorful tin cans that once contained a myriad of products were nailed to the walls to create an undulating surface. Each one was a different size or shape or color. They had held cookies or biscuits or fruitcake or crackers, and their variety reflected the ever-changing taste of generations of designers and consumers.

Dad and I ordered coffee. I took some extra sugar packets and put them in my purse so Dad would have sugar for his coffee the next morning. I felt a little guilty, but not enough to put the packets back. We finished breakfast and asked the waitress directions to the closest grocery store.

"Albertson's," she said. "It's real close. Are you visiting?"

"Yes, we're here from Chicago to go to the Hammesfahr Neurological Institute."

"Oh," she said, unimpressed. Although the Institute was right in town, she had obviously never heard of it.

"Can you tell me how to get to the store?"

"Sure. Go up the street, left turn on Druid Street to Missouri and turn right. Albertson's is on the left a few blocks farther." The next block over was Druid Street. That was the address of the Hammesfahr Neurological Institute where we were going this afternoon. It was close by.

We finished breakfast and took off making a short detour to drive directly past the two-story white building that housed the Institute. There was a parking lot in front of the old mansion, on what once must have been a lawn. Two colonnades rose on either side of the front entry. There was a ramp for wheelchairs on one side. Four wooden steps led up to the porch, where a rattan love seat with blue and white cushions and sat empty. The parking lot was full. There was no sign of people.

"This is it, Dad. We're going right past it."

"I know." He sounded tense. "Maybe they will want to pass me up when I get there."

"You'll probably be passable." I played with the word. "Don't worry so much. They are going to want to see you."

"You never know. I may not be a candidate for this treatment." Dad smiled, but he sounded doubtful.

"You must feel a little more confident, because you're letting me go grocery shopping."

"Just one day's worth," he said. "We're not making any commitments."

Other doctors' offices, also housed in old mansions, surrounded the Institute. There were some small massage therapy businesses and then the street became residential. We drove silently on, each with our own skeptical thoughts.

I hate grocery stores. For years, I took three children to the grocery store and bought a host of generic items. I took a calculator and did price comparisons between

different brands of toilet paper. I read labels to avoid foods
that my oldest son, Rollins, who was allergic to many foods,
couldn't eat. On a single mother's budget, I bought two full
carts every time. Women at the checkout stand would
marvel. Those mammoth all-day-shopping excursions
involved trip after trip up two flights of stairs carting the
groceries from my double-parked station wagon to the
kitchen in the far back of the apartment, and ended with
hours spent putting the food away.

It was difficult to concentrate at Albertson's. Every
other thought was about the event that hung just out of reach
a few hours later. We bought cereal, milk, bananas, bread,
mustard, lettuce, sliced turkey and coffee. When we got
through the line, I decided that we had better get some pasta
and tomato sauce for supper that night, so I went through the
line a second time. When we got back to the motel we
discovered that we did not have dishwashing soap, napkins
or salad dressing, and I knew that we would have to go back
to the store again. I even forgot something that was on my
grocery list. My thoughts were on the Institute, not the
groceries.

I left Dad taking a nap and went out to the motel
swimming pool. I counted twelve strokes from one side of
the pool to the other. I counted twenty-four seconds for each
lap. I swam one hundred laps. I tried not to think of anything
but numbers while I waited for the time to pass until our 2
PM appointment.

Back in the room, I got Dad into the shower and
washed his hair and body. I had not seen him naked since the
previous year, when he'd come to visit Steve and me. His
skin was like a young child's, fine and smooth and white. My
dermatologist had said that my skin was already badly
damaged, but Dad's back was young and soft. He'd always
disliked the sun and kept his shirt on. I should have followed
his example. He seemed to be aging in sections. His face

looked his eighty-two years, but his back could have been eighteen.

Tension mounted as I fixed lunch for Dad. My stomach was too tight to eat, but I drank a glass of water as I cleared up the dishes. I took a shower, dressed, and assembled all of the paperwork for the doctor. At one-twenty I said, "Let's go. If we get there early we can wait in the office."

There was little traffic, but we managed to hit every red light. Finally, we turned into the driveway.

The front door opened on two rooms, once parlors. They were filled with people, some of them in wheelchairs and braces, some looking perfectly normal. The floors were covered with oriental rugs. Bookshelves were piled with paperbacks and magazines. Antiques filled the rooms. Love seats and high-backed upholstered chairs stood in all the available spaces.

Talking filled the air. One of the men pointed out a picture called "Never Give Up." A frog was half way down the throat of a heron, but hanging on for his life with his arms around the heron's neck and his feet braced out too wide for the bird to swallow.

Dad and I felt like the frog, about to be consumed. I just didn't know whether we would be consumed by the doctors or by the disease. The man gave us a photocopy of the picture and I smiled ruefully as I put it in the clear plastic folder that held my father's medical history. Every time I picked up the folder I would see it.

A young girl with long brown hair greeted us and asked Dad to sign in on a list at the door. She asked me to sign in, as well. She looked nervous.

"My name is Summer," she said. "Summer Rose Wright."

"And mine is Robin," I said.

"Oh, I get it… robin-summer."

"Was your mother a hippie?" I asked.

"No. She's born again. Her name is Rose Wright. I'm named after her."

I named my daughter Jolie Arleen after my mother. That wasn't too unusual. But Summer's name gave me all kinds of playful thoughts. I thought of Summer Rising in Mrs. Wright's pregnancy. Or Summer Rose, right? Or Rose Wright, born again as Summer. I couldn't help myself. My dad had plagued us with this silly word banter until he had had his stroke and didn't think so well. He had to be having a good day for him to attempt it since the stroke.

Summer left us to go to the desk. In a moment she was back, all business. "Would you come into the office?" She led us to the sunroom of the old mansion, where her desk, chair, copy machine, and filing cabinets filled the space. The big desk made her seem small and vulnerable. Her voice quavered as she sat and stated, "The fee for this procedure is $5,000. No insurance policy will cover it. Medicare will not cover it. Will you be paying by Visa, Master Charge or cashier's check?"

That got that out front. There were no ifs, ands, or buts. You want to go any further, put your money on the table. No going back. This was it. Make a commitment now. Dad handed over his Visa card. She gave us a little receipt, handwritten in the kind of receipt book I'd used for students to pay school fees.

"What about a whole bill?" I asked. "My father has several insurance companies that ought to pay this bill but they won't on the basis of this little piece of paper."

Summer smiled. "He'll get a detailed bill in the mail."

"Can't I get it here? I am not going home with him, and I won't be there to help him file the claims."

"I don't know," she said. "I'm new here. This is only my second day. I'll ask when I get upstairs." She sounded a little panicked, like my teenage students when I called on them and they didn't know the answer.

We returned to the lobby and sat down. A nurse came in carrying a big easel with white paper on it. "My name is Sharon Chickoree," she said, as she set the easel up in front of us.

Chickoree, I thought. Another odd name.

She handed us a blue three-ring binder with a picture of the Institute on the front. "If you open your folder, you can follow along."

The binder began with a section that described the major players at the institute. The first picture and biography were of Dr. Hammesfahr. He was handsome and young.

"His work in Stroke, Brain Injury, Learning Disabilities, Autism, and Dyslexia has broken new ground. He was one of the very few, extra brilliant students selected for admission into Northwestern University's Medical School directly from high school." I remembered that special program from my days of teaching. The school selected promising students and enrolled them directly into medical school. They took honors classes.

He graduated in 1982 with a degree in neurology. He did his residency at the Medical College of Virginia. "This therapy also garnered him the 1999 nomination for the Nobel Prize in Medicine and Physiology. One of the very few nominations worldwide, his was of the highest order, a Congressional nomination. He was published on the web site of the Nobel Prize at the Karolinski Institute."

I began to feel more secure about this doctor and his Institute. The information went on, "A study finds that ninety percent of his patients show improvement within the first ten days of treatment."

"Great earrings," Sharon said, pointing to my smashed beer bottle caps that had been made into yellow earrings. "That beer, Caribe, is made in Trinidad, where I'm from."

Obviously, the woman had great taste and was destined to be our friend. How easily won I am by the smallest bit of flattery.

She gave us a lecture on what to do and what not to do, pointing out the lists in the Blue Book. The directions were very precise. There were lots of, "If your blood pressure goes down." The details in the Blue Book made things seem more complicated but also had answers for many questions.

The following is a list of Do Not behavior:

No smoking for you, your spouse or anyone around you

No grapefruit juice – it changes the potency of the medications

No skipping meals or the required water

No diet sweeteners in any form

No decongestants

No hot tubs, saunas or exposure to heat

No aerobic exercises

No substituting medicines

No chocolate

No alcohol

No caffeine (maybe six ounces of coffee if you're desperate)

No Viagra - it will kill you

And the DO behavior:

Drink 64 ounces of water a day before 4pm. (Really. She means it!)

Drink cranberry juice

Take your blood pressure before breakfast and before dinner

Take your pills after meals

See your family doctor monthly

Be positive and upbeat

Dad said he could live with that. Summer introduced us to a stocky man in a white coat. This was Dr. B. A.

Raines. I peeked at his brief biography. He had been president of the Florida Medical Society, and his grin was so big you could easily see why. He had dark hair and a square face and body. He moved quickly and spoke just as fast.

"Did you watch the videotape?" he asked.

"Yes, we did," Dad said.

"Let me explain it again," Dr. Raines began. "We use common vasodilators to open up vessels that have been narrowed since the stroke. These vessels will bring blood back to parts of the brain that have been deprived of it. That begins the self-healing process." He drew a dark spot on a pad of paper, and four concentric circles around it.

"Think of it like peeling an onion. Artery healing begins with the outer circle. This area is most the accessible and the first to be affected by the medications. If there are injuries to the nerves in this section of the brain, improvement is often seen in the first few weeks of treatment. If the injuries are in the second circle, the repair work is seen in the first six months. Healing in the third circle is much slower, sometimes taking years. The center dark spot is the totally ruined brain at the epicenter of the stroke. It may never heal."

This theory explained why some patients had recovery in the first hours after taking the medication. It explained why the treatment seemed so miraculous. Dad signed a paper that said that there were no guarantees.

Sharon returned. "Now, if you feel better, don't go starting any exercise programs," she cautioned. "Some people feel so good they think that they can go out and roller blade and they fall. That would not be good."

I looked at the people in the wheelchairs and imagined them rollerblading and laughed. "I had high hopes that Dad would be able to go surfing soon. He's never done that before, but since you warned me, I will lower my expectations. Maybe just a little soft shoe and a song." I teased her, but I hoped that I would be able to dance with my Daddy again.

She laughed.

"You are invited to the Clearwater Yacht Club for an Education Session that runs from two-thirty to four-thirty on Tuesdays and Thursdays. There's lots of food there - sandwiches, meatballs, fruit, cookies, and water."

The meeting had already started when we arrived at the Yacht Club. Beside the front door was a tub filled with many, many bottles of water. Each patient must drink sixty-four ounces of water a day because water affects the absorption rate of the medications. Caregivers also drank water, out of compassion and guilt. That seemed like an enormous amount of water and everyone struggled to get it down.

At the front of the room, Dr. Hammesfahr was forcefully describing the physiology of a stroke. He looked too young to know as much as I thought he should know, but he also looked very strong and confident. He had unusually bright blue, clearly intelligent eyes. I trusted this man for no reason but that I could look deep into his soul through those eyes. They were Shakespeare eyes. Angel eyes. He looked as though he knew the secret to recovery and the faster he could spread it around, the better it would be for the whole world. His appearance of self-confidence was extraordinary. He knew the answers to every question these patients had about their strokes. He spoke very fast.

"It doesn't matter how you got the stroke, whether a bleed or a clot, the results are the same. Blood vessels are constricted, cutting off the flow of blood to the brain and causing the symptoms you know as tight muscles, loss of speech, and so on."

I looked around at all the caregivers in the room. One wife sat with her hand placed on her invalid husband's hands. He had folded his hands across his stomach in order to hold down the arm affected by the stroke. She patted them softly and he looked up at her and smiled. Their love was palpable.

Daughters and sons sat beside afflicted mothers and fathers, taking notes and asking questions about their individual cases. The room was filled with compassion. These people loved each other and they all had hope of recovery.

"Each case is unique," Dr. Hammesfahr continued. "Each case needs different medications at different doses. That is why you must check your blood pressure twice every day. If it goes out of your acceptable range, call your doctor immediately."

Each is unique, I thought. Just like the tin cans in the restaurant where we'd had breakfast that morning. Just like my Dad.

The physical therapist, Diane Hartley, spoke next. She was a short woman with cropped blonde hair, who exuded pep and energy. She described an accident in which she had injured her spine and used Dr. Hammesfahr's therapy to recover.

"I thought that once I was back to normal, I could stop taking the medication," she said. "So I stopped. The first week I was fine. The second week the symptoms began to reappear. Let me advise you. Do not stop taking your medicine. You must take this medicine for the rest of your life."

Finally, Dr. Allen P. Gimon, the good looking educational psychologist spoke. He was young, stocky, and well dressed. He handed out little thermometers. I thought that was a good sign, as I was freezing in the high volume air conditioning. "Hold these between your thumb and your first finger. If you are relaxed, and your blood vessels are dilated, your temperature should go up to around ninety-three degrees. I looked at mine. It stayed right at eighty degrees. Stress aplenty. "How is yours?" I whispered to Dad.

"Ninety-two," he whispered back.

"You had the stroke, Dad. How come I'm the one with constricted blood vessels?"

The meeting broke up and I gathered our empty plates. "What should I do with these?" I asked a woman in a blue Hammesfahr golf shirt.

"I'll take them," she said. "Are you new?"

"Yes. I'm from Chicago and Dad is from Rock Island."

"I'm from Chicago, around Belmont Avenue. My name is Donna." She smiled and her blue eyes crinkled. Like Sharon, she also exuded energy, optimism, and positive vibrations.

"I live on West Sheridan Road," I said. "Belmont is just a few blocks south."

"My son just moved to that neighborhood. Have you seen Sue?"

"Yes. There are long lines to see that dinosaur, but we went early one morning and got in after only twenty minutes. I like the dancing brontosaurus outside the Field Museum, too."

"Isn't she spectacular? Even though we really don't know if she is a she." Donna rattled on with a great deal of cheer. "I wrote a children's poem about that dinosaur."

"I'd love to read it. I used to teach writing. This is my father, Woody Robinson." Dad rose and extended his right hand with the curved fingers, while he held his cane with his left hand.

"I don't really have a hand any more. I'm sorry."

She touched his clawed fingers. "Don't be sorry. We're going to fix that. That's what we do here," she said.

Suddenly, my eyes filled with tears. I had to blink to be able to see. Donna noticed and touched my arm. "Honey, he's going to get better. Everyone gets better here."

"I can't believe it. I want to, but it seems so impossible. Whenever I think that it could really happen I get emotional and cry," I whispered and turned away so my father would not see me.

Donna patted my arm. "You'll soon have something to sing about."

"Dad, do you have something to sing about?" I asked, turning back. "My dad was a singer during the big band days." I bragged to Donna.

He began whispering hoarsely.

"It ain't necessarily so,
The things that you're liable
To read in the Bible
They ain't necessarily so."

Donna joined in, filling in words where Dad forgot them. They reflected exactly what I was thinking. It ain't necessarily so.

We rode back from Clearwater Beach to our motel in silence, each immersed in our own thoughts. On the way across the causeway there were two huge white herons standing in the middle of a grassy field.

"Look Dad! You can tell Mom thinks we are doing the right thing. See her birds? She's with us." Mom knew when to give us some of her style of encouragement. We both felt calmer.

Soon after Mother died, Steve and I took a vacation on Virgin Gorda, an island in the British West Indies. Our hotel room stood on stilts high above the ground and overlooked a steep grassy incline down to a small beach. The incline was full of trees that enveloped the porch that wrapped around the room. One day I sat out there to read and was surrounded by hundreds of small dark birds. They flitted from tree to tree, making a huge ruckus. It was impossible to concentrate on my book. They stayed there, cackling away, until I thought about my mother. Then they left all at once. That was the first time that I understood that Mother was trying to communicate with me through birds. It sounds strange, but I knew it without a doubt.

The Greek playwright, Sophocles, wrote about Teiresius, the blind soothsayer, getting divination from the birds. Uncle Remus had a bluebird on his shoulder. Walt Disney's Cinderella had birds that helped her get dressed. I had a good grounding in history and myth for this sort of thing. Getting messages from birds was an old tradition. After that, I vowed to remember to look to birds with great care for mother's counsel.

10
Fear of Failure
Wednesday, October 4
Day Two

We began Wednesday with an appointment to measure Dad's physical abilities before he began therapy. The physical therapist's office was ready to take us when we arrived at nine. I filled out forms and Dad paid the bill, putting another $300 on his Visa card.

Alex, the physical therapist, began by asking a series of questions focusing on Dad's ability to move.

"First close your eyes. Can you feel this?" Alex rubbed his finger along the bottom of Dad's clenched right hand. "Point to where I am touching with your left hand." Dad shook his head no. "How about here?" Alex said as he moved the tiny metal rod around on dad's paralyzed right hand.

Dad missed identifying *all* of the places that Alex touched.

"I can't feel anything at all," he finally confessed.

When Alex closed Dad's right hand and asked him to mimic the motion with his left hand, Dad did the opposite and extended the fingers of his left hand. He definitely flunked 'hand.'

His right foot had more feeling than his right hand, however. Dad could tell where Alex touched him and where he pricked him with a pin. Later, I would realize the significance of this.

Emily came into the room to do the Ease-of-Movement test, a gauge of dad's ability to move in space. Dad walked back and forth across the room while a video camera recorded his movement. Next, Alex asked him to raise his arms above his head and then to cross them over as far right and then as far left as he could. Alex put a wooden block on the floor and asked Dad to pick it up with his good hand.

While Dad was seated in a chair, Alex asked him to point his left foot which worked pretty well. When he was asked to point his right foot it jerked spastically in various uncontrollable directions instead of pointing.

Dad stood up again and Alex asked him to turn around.

"I get dizzy," Dad said as he awkwardly took uneven steps to make the circle.

Finally, Alex asked him to try to balance on one foot. He stood for seven seconds on his left leg. He could not balance at all on his right foot.

"See, Dad. Everything you needed to know in life you did learn in kindergarten." I thought of the small book popular several years ago. Walking, turning, standing, sitting, bending, and balance: children spend the first few years of their lives learning to do all of these things. Dad had lost the ability to do them. He was eighty-two.

It was ten o'clock when we left the physical therapist's office and drove the few blocks back to the Institute.

"I was all thumbs," Dad said.

"Actually, I thought you did better than you usually do. Were you really trying hard?"

"Yeah, I was."

"Maybe you shouldn't have tried so hard this time and then you would do better the next time they test you. That would make it look like you are improving."

"I don't need to look better. I need to be better." Dad adjusted the air conditioning with his left hand.

"So, I suppose cheating won't work?"

"There's no point to it."

We pulled into the Institute parking lot. Dad eased himself out of the car and slammed the door. We climbed the ramp to the front door and I held it open for Dad. Opening a door and holding a cane were mutually exclusive things for him. He had to shift his cane to his bad hand and keep his balance while he used his good hand to pull the door. Often, that resulted in his cane dropping and rattling across the floor. If his cane fell, he was confronted with the problem of bending over and picking up the cane, without falling. He would grope for it with the damaged fingers that refused to fold neatly, as he propped himself against the door with his good hand.

Everything is more difficult for a stroke victim.

Sharon took us immediately into the ultrasound room. Dad sat in a big recliner chair while Sharon took his blood pressure. It was 105/72.

"You are going to have to buy a blood pressure machine if you don't have one," she said. "You'll need to take your blood pressure morning and evening, at the same time every day. Record it in the little blue book we gave you. You can get the machine at Wal-Mart. Bring it in to the office and we will calibrate it for you." She gave us the brand names of several good machines. Next, Sharon introduced us to Debbie Powers, our ultrasound technician.

Debbie was a cute redhead with tiny curls all over her head and a big smile. Her biography in the blue folder said that she loved working at the Institute because of all the 'miracles' that happen to the patients there. We were certainly in the realm of the sunshine people. I wondered if employees were instructed to be extra cheerful or if they were that way because they were working in this hopeful place. Maybe the Institute only hired good-natured people. Debbie began explaining what she was going to do.

"Could I go to the bathroom before you start these tests?" Dad asked. He had never ending bladder problems and he had been trying to drink more water, which made things worse. He liked to plan ahead.

"Absolutely." She pushed the recliner chair into a vertical position and Dad struggled to get out of it.

When Dad again sat in the reclining wing back chair, Debbie showed him the electrodes she was going to attach to his body for the ultrasound that would measure his heartbeat. I saw fuzzy pictures appear on her screen. After she printed these pictures, she changed his electrodes to the carotid arteries that ran down the left and the right sides of his neck. The screen was fuzzy and floaters continually crossed it, but sometimes I could see actual artery walls. I could even see the white plaque along the edges of the walls.

"Okay. You're done," Debbie said as she attached the pictures she had printed on to Dad's file. "Ill just show these to the doctor."

I gathered my information-laden purse and bag of medical records to leave. Just as we were opening the front door, Debbie came rushing after us. "Could you wait a minute?" she asked. "The doctor is still checking the ultrasound pictures.

"Sure," Dad said. He sat on the rattan loveseat on the sun porch. I took the chair beside him.

The door opened again and a spry, blonde in a pale pink sweater set came out. "Could I sit here?" she asked, indicating the seat beside Dad. She was tiny like my mother and she had clear translucent skin without any trace of Florida tan.

Dad smiled. He was always pleased to be near a pretty woman. "Be my guest."

"My name is Robin and this is my Dad, Woody."

"I'm Angela."

"We just got here and we haven't started therapy yet. We're a little worried. How long have you been coming here?" I asked.

"This is my second week. I'm from Pensacola."

"Have you seen any improvement since you got here?" Dad asked.

"Yes, my arm is much better." She fingered her right hand. "It was much tighter last week. I'm walking better, too."

"I hope that happens to me," Dad said.

"It probably will. Almost everyone gets better here." Angela encouraged him. I watched him admiring her.

"I have to stay here most of the day because they can't get my blood pressure stabilized. It doesn't matter whether I sit here at the Institute or back in the motel. I came here alone."

"I hope that doesn't happen to me," Dad said.

"It probably won't."

Debbie came out with several pieces of paper. "We can't see your left artery clearly enough. The doctor wants you to get an MRI. Here is a prescription for Horizon Diagnostic Center. It's a few blocks down on Avenue D."

"I know where that is," I said, taking the papers. I had seen Avenue D when we missed the turn on to Druid Street that morning.

"Call them for an appointment and tell them that you are coming from Dr. Hammesfahr. They'll get you in right away."

I pulled out my cell phone and made the call.

"We have an opening tomorrow afternoon at three-thirty," the receptionist said. "Can you make it then?"

"Absolutely," I said. I didn't know how long the appointment would be at the Institute so I checked with

Sharon to make sure that we could make a one o'clock appointment and then a three-thirty appointment.

"We can't proceed with medications until we get the MRI back so that is the most important appointment now. I don't think you will have any problem with the schedule and if you do, we'll just change your appointment at the Institute to a later time," she said.

Tomorrow would be a full day. Dad had three appointments: one with a physician at Dr. Hammesfahr's Institute, one with the educational psychologist, and one with the MRI machine.

"See you tomorrow," Dad said to Angela as we left the porch.

We headed to the Wal-Mart to get Dad some shorts so I wouldn't have to do laundry every other day, and to buy a blood pressure machine. Next to Wal-Mart was a Dollar Store. We went to it first.

I loved Dollar Stores. I always found things that I desperately needed, even though I was not usually aware of that need until I actually saw the items. In this store, I purchased a large plastic tray, two plastic glasses to use around the pool, and a box of magnetic alphabet letters for the refrigerator. I didn't really need the alphabet letters, but I knew I could have fun with them.

Then we traipsed over to Wal-Mart to see if we could get a blood pressure machine that Dad could take home with him. The machine was $70. He didn't try on the shorts I picked out, but I measured his waist and it was forty-seven inches. I bought size forty-six and forty-eight.

When, we got back to the motel, Dad sat down in front of the TV to watch CNBC. He dozed almost immediately. I fixed dinner.

My sister called after we ate dinner.

"How did you get the records from County Hospital?" I asked. "I'm amazed."

Lia spoke matter-of-factly, but I heard the pride in her voice. "When I called, I asked who it was on the phone. It turned out to be a woman whose kids had been students of mine in Mom's nursery school for years. They'd also taken swimming lessons from me for four summers straight. She owed me one."

"You are one terrific sister. Dad was worried about the Institute not taking him as a patient. I'm sure those records will help a lot."

"Let me talk to him," she said. I handed over the phone.

He smiled. "You two made up?" he asked me.

I grinned back, "I think so."

11
Ups and Downs
Thursday, October 5
Day Three

Dad didn't have an appointment at the Institute until eleven-thirty. This one was with the doctor who would actually be determining his medications. I was impatient, but the morning went quickly. I took Dad's blood pressure, fed him breakfast, gave him a shower and helped him dress. Dressing was always a problem for Dad, especially trying to put on his socks with only his left hand functioning. We tried two pairs before we got socks that would slide easily onto his feet. I swam for thirty-minutes, showered, and dressed. Then it was time to leave for the Institute.

"You're going to like this day, Dad. You get to spend an hour talking about yourself with one of the Institute doctors. Not many people get to devote an entire hour to their egos."

"I'm paying for it," he said sardonically.

I tried to joke. "You probably want to discuss your love life. Regrettably, the doctor is not interested in your love life. He's only interested in medical things."

"What love life?" Dad said, as we pulled into the parking lot and looked for a spot under a tree.

An aide rushed out on the porch to help Dad up the three steps into the Institute. It was hard to find a place to sit because people in wheel chairs, and with various braces on their arms and legs, packed the waiting room. Nurses, aides, doctors, and other cheery persons moved quickly among all the wheelchairs and braces, dispensing water and advice about such diverse subjects as blood pressure and good restaurants.

I had recently seen a play produced by Lookingglass Theater in Chicago called "Metamorphosis." The director, David Catlin, created a very physical theater piece from a short story by Kafka in which a middle-aged salesman, Gregor, went to bed a normal human being and awoke transformed into a cockroach. He could not speak. He could not use his hands. His arms and legs had tensed into frozen angles. He was trapped in the hard cased body of an insect. He was deformed; a monster that reminded me of the stroke victims sitting in front of us at Dr. Hammesfahr's office.

When Gregor finally emerged from his room, which was a glass box suspended above the stage, he walked on stilts that were held on by braces. His arms were attached to crutches by braces. He walked painfully and slowly, his distorted body supported by his four braced limbs. The actor who played the part, Larry DiStasi, had transformed himself into a grotesque and I pitied his muscles at the end of a performance because they had been held in awkward contraction for the several hours in which he performed in the play each night. But he didn't have to live in a body that didn't work. He changed himself into an insect with the use of the same braces and support equipment used by stroke victims on a daily basis. My father's muscles had been in contraction every waking hour for eight years, ever since he had the stroke. His pain was beyond my knowing.

Before turning into a monster, the salesman, Gregor, his father, and another actor were engaged in a "dance of work." They put their bowler hats on with their dark suits and picked up their briefcases. They marched three abreast, in their bare feet, to the front of the stage, stomping their feet, taking tiny steps, then slamming their briefcases on the ground and picking them up again. All the actions were an imitation of the repetitive day-to-day work that most of us experience. This powerful dance of their unaware lives was almost as terrifying as Gregor's transformation into a cockroach.

Our daily lives went on for us in this same unaware, repetitive fashion until a stroke shattered our family's routine. We had to cope with enormous changes because of Mother's stroke and then Dad's catastrophic brain hemorrhage. The changes necessitated by the stroke were as catastrophic to the entire family as the stroke was to Dad's brain. Many people in the Institute's waiting room were much worse than my father.

Gregor's family, his mother, father, and sister were horrified. His father refused to acknowledge or to look at him. His mother eventually tried to enter his room, only to be frightened away by the appearance of the cockroach. It was left to his sister to feed and water him, a task that she did at four in the morning in order not to disturb the other members of the household. Gregor hid under the bed to spare his sister so that she didn't have to look at him when she put out his food and water.

My sister was Mother and Dad's primary caretaker. She had the responsibility of cleaning, feeding, bathing, combing the hair, brushing the teeth, and if necessary, wiping the bottoms of her parents. I watched the caregivers who were here at the Institute in the room sitting among the stroke patients with Dad and me. Like my sister, they were bringing them water, interpreting instructions and conversations, and waiting. The caregivers were as trapped in their roles as the patients were trapped in their stroke ridden bodies.

Gregor, the cockroach, could not have been more frightening than this room full of people encased in plastic and metal. He could not have changed more suddenly than the strokes changed these patients. One day they could talk and walk and the next day they couldn't. And many had had no hope for recovery during the five or ten or twenty years since their strokes.

Some families choose to send their stroke patients to a care center to put them out of sight. Others struggle with help at home and some brave souls nurse their patients, their loved ones, alone. I wondered what amazing set of circumstances had brought each of these people to this waiting room.

Donna, jovial as always, came by and schmoozed a little. She wore the classic blue golf shirt and the ready smile that all the auxiliary staff wore.

"Will you sing at the Yacht Club next week?" She put her arm around Dad's shoulders. Since Mother died, not many people touched my father.

"I don't remember the words to songs anymore." He shook his head in a firm no.

"Those words will come back to you pretty soon," Donna said confidently.

"Why don't you practice?" I suggested, trying to make the situation positive. "Life is just a bowl of cherries...," I began.

Dad and Donna joined in, Dad coming in the middle of the lines, letting us take the lead.

"Don't make it serious,"
Life's too mysterious,
You work, you save, you worry so,
But you can't take your dough when you go, go, go,
So keep repeating it's the berries
And live and laugh at it all."

The roomful of caregivers applauded. The patients brightened up, but held their affected arms tightly against their chests, unable to clap with clenched hands. Finally, even Dad smiled.

We waited. Forty-five minutes later, Sharon, the nurse, took us into an office that looked as though it had once been a dining room to the house.

"The doctor will be in to see you here," she said.

"We would like to see Dr. Hammesfahr," I said.

"He usually sees the more difficult cases," Sharon said. "You'll like all of our doctors." She took Dad's blood pressure, 137/80.

"I guess we're not a difficult case," I said.

"Not yet. Please take off your shoes and socks," she directed.

We struggled to take off his socks again.

This room had an oriental rug and a table, but its most notable object was the long human spine hanging from a rack near the fireplace. A clock on the mantelpiece said eight o'clock. It was twelve-fifteen. Two leather chairs faced a table. There was a box of Kleenex on the desk. Behind the desk were a computer, TV/VCR, and a white porcelain head with phrenology markings. Quite a contrast, computers and phrenology!

Phrenology was a bizarre nineteenth century science of interpreting the brain by feeling the bumps on the outside of the head. Its inventor, Franz Gall, had the right idea. Different parts of the brain do control different actions and thoughts in the body. The problem with his theory was that science in the 1800s did not have the equipment to go inside the brain and map its activity, so Gall decided he could tell what was happening inside the brain by feeling the bumps on the outside. The head was divided into sections labeled Wondering, Humor, Intuitiveness, and Hope on the right side, and Egotism, Morals, and Selfishness on the left. Needless to say, belief in this pseudo science did not last long. The piece of statuary was perfect in a neurologist's office. It served to remind me how far medicine had come in the last hundred years.

There was also a plastic model of a whole brain and beside it another plastic brain that was cut in half. An ironic item, considering how many patients came into that office with half a functioning brain. On the wall were Dr. Hammesfahr's diplomas: Medicine from Northwestern University in 1982, Residency in Neurology at the College of Virginia in 1988, and Board Certification in 1992. Reassuring. Solid.

Dad was whispering something to himself. If I hadn't known him better, I would have said it was a prayer.

"What are you whispering?" I asked.

"I was singing," he said. "The Green-eyed Dragon."

I remembered that song. Dad had sung it for years. Mrs. Polly, Dad's voice teacher in the 1930s, had given him the patter song to improve his diction.

"I wanted to see if my mind would remember all the words." He said it as though his mind was a separate entity over which he had no control. Dad had separated his mind from the rest of his self-worth, as though it was a foreign object, to be tested and measured as he was trained to do as a psychologist.

Dad had sung it to me so often that I knew part of the song.

"Beware!

Take care!

Of the green-eyed dragon with the thirteen tails,

He'll feed, with greed,

On little boys, puppy dogs, and big fat snails."

I wondered whether Dad thought he was a little boy, a puppy dog, or a big fat snail. I wondered if he thought the doctor was the green-eyed dragon.

"Did your mind remember the words?" I asked.

"Not at the end. The end I couldn't remember. I almost got to the end, though. It's been years since I sang that song."

I didn't know whether he meant sang it professionally, or sang it to me. He had sung it to me often, but evidently he didn't remember.

We waited some more. At that point we were an hour behind schedule.

At twelve-twenty, Dad had to urinate. Sharon pointed out the bathroom. I pointed out to her that we were due at Dr. Gimon's office at one and the directions said it took fifteen minutes to get there.

"Go ahead," she advised. "We will reschedule this appointment for tomorrow. We have to have all of the reports before we can start medication anyway. We can't do anything until we get the MRI." She left the room.

There was nothing we could do but go on to the next appointment.

"I guess I'm not important enough," Dad said.

"Of course you are important," I said. "They're busy."

"Too busy to make time for me," he concluded. "So much for talking about me."

I put Dad's shoes back on. We gave up and left the socks off. This was Florida, after all. I stuffed them in my purse.

We headed south on Fort Harrison Avenue to the educational psychologist's office. Strip mall after strip mall of offices and stores lined the road. The sun was hot on our windows and the air conditioner was working overtime.

"Now they are going to test your brain," I said.

"If I have one anymore. I used to have a brain," Dad lamented. "You know, Robin, I taught a class called Tests and Measurements for years. Do you think I should tell them that?"

"If you don't, I will."

The office was at the back of a complex of one-story buildings. Its door opened onto a long staircase. "If I have to climb those stairs I'm going to be mad," Dad whispered.

The elderly receptionist smiled at us. "Mr. Rush?" she asked.

"No. Dr. Robinson," I answered, emphasizing the doctor. She checked her schedule.

"He's not due here until two-thirty."

"He's got an MRI at three-thirty. Two-thirty won't work." I showed her the three weeks of pre-scheduled appointments that had been given us in the blue three-ring binder. It clearly stated that the appointment was for one o'clock.

"Let's see what I can do." She went down a long hall into the back of the office. In a moment another woman came out. "We must have gotten our wires crossed," she said. "The doctor is going over to The Oaks to administer these psychological tests to the patients in wheelchairs who are staying there. That way they won't have to put them in vans and haul them over here. You can talk to Timothy."

That was nice, but I didn't understand who Timothy was and what their scheduling had to do with us. Dad charged another $590 to his Visa card at the front desk. I got handed the forms to fill out.

"Timothy will see you next," the receptionist reassured us.

Timothy was a young Asian man with a nervous smile. He took my father into a back room while I filled out forms. When I came into the room Dad was busy tapping on an electric board with his left hand. Timothy sat beside him.

On the wall were two diplomas listing Timothy' name as Manivong. "Do you have a doctorate in Educational Psychology?" I asked.

"I'm writing my dissertation now," he said.

"My father taught graduate students like you in Tests and Measurements classes."

"I've administered these tests many times," Dad
added. "I'll remember the answers."

"Where are you from, Mr. Manivong?" I tried to
pronounce his name as a test for myself in phonic
recognition. Teaching in the inner city meant that I always
had students with unpronounceable names from all over the
world.

"Laos. I came here when I was ten."

Timothy and Dad started the next test, a "What's
Missing from This Picture?" exercise. Dad did well until
they came to a picture of a person walking a dog on the
beach. He said that the dog needed a leash, (which it did, at
least on Chicago beaches) instead of saying that there were
no dog footprints in the sand. He was at the mercy of
Timothy, the test master.

He went on to take tests that measured concentration,
motor speed, attention, orientation, hemisphere dominance,
short-term memory, processing, fluency, and IQ.

During the test for word memory Timothy said five
words and asked Dad to repeat them. "What did you say?"
My father balked at the list. "I didn't understand you."

"I can't repeat them."

I was also trying to decipher the last two words
which sounded like "sadow" and "bubbow," with Timothy's
Asian accent. I watched him pronounce the words when he
read the list a second time. His mouth formed the shape for a
"ow" sound, but what he meant was "le." He was trying to
say saddle and bubble. My father said, "shadow" and "I don't
know the last one."

Then Timothy told us how well Dad had done on
each test. It was a little disconcerting to have his infirmities
measured and quantified. Timothy said things like, "Time
was pretty good, but you made some errors." Not great for
Dad's beleaguered self-esteem, even if true.

By the time we left the office, both of us were feeling
down. My shoulders were hunched way up around my neck.

Dad looked at me. "Take a deep breath and let it out slowly," he ordered, giving me his version of the Cosmic Sigh. "And drop your shoulders." I did and it helped.

I had packed a light lunch that morning, and we found a little park beside a lake, where we could eat. "See that Historical Society?" I pointed to a building next to the parking lot. "That's the kind of place mom would have made us stop at when I was little."

"I remember." Dad was struggling across the grass with his cane. "She always wanted to know more, to know everything, like you do. I miss her."

"I know," I said quietly. "I do too."

"Do you think I'll ever see her again?" he asked. Dad had always been an agnostic, professing not to know about life after death, but I heard the plea in his voice for a heaven in which he could return to his life with my mother. I couldn't answer.

Finally I said, "You know Mom, she's busy mapping the universe and making duplicate copies for her report to Archangel Michael and the head of the Wing Department." He laughed a bit.

"She's doing research," I went on, wanting him to laugh a little more. "Remember when she gave the old pill bottles with child-proof tops to the nursery school kids?"

"Yeah, it took them about three minutes to open those bottles."

"That was a research project for some class she was taking," I said as I handed him his sandwich. We sat silently chewing and remembering as we watched the water.

Mother loved to walk in the woods. She could identify all the Midwestern wild flowers and trees. She knew all the birds. She knew how to be silent in the woods like we were beside the pond water. Often we watched her paint or sketch in her spiral bound watercolor books.

Cruelly, the stroke first took her ability to walk. When we took her to the woods, she cried for the things that she could no longer do. A wheelchair does not push easily on a woodland path. The bumpy ride was painful to her frail body's bones. From then on we went only to places that were paved and handicapped accessible.

In the early summer we pushed her out to the swimming pool and dangled her feet off her wheelchair's foot props. Two useless appendages swung in mid-air and splashed into the cool water. She wiggled the left one, sending small ripples over the pale blue surface. The right one hung without sensation, ankle deep in the water. I was swimming my laps, pausing to tickle her non-feeling toes when I noticed her skin. The water had turned big sections of the bottom of her feet pasty white. Old dead skin had accumulated between her toes and on her heels. She was decaying from the bottom up.

After my swim, I sat on the edge of the pool and pulled Mom's feet out of the water. I scraped the layers of scummy skin off the bottoms and rubbed them dry with a towel and her pink feet began to emerge. We had hired a staff of practical nurses who bathed her daily, but I guess that her feet were not their priority.

My mother began teaching in 1934, when she was sixteen years old, in a one-room schoolhouse in the sand hills of northeast Nebraska. In the 1960s, she started the first nursery school in the little Illinois college town where Dad taught. She spent many years teaching hundreds of children to swim in our backyard pool. Her second stroke took her ability to speak, silencing her inquiring mind forever after. Not that my sister and I didn't believe we knew exactly what she was thinking. Daughters who had watched their mother for fifty years knew what her smallest glance meant. But my mother was always full of surprises.

We would think that we had her pegged and she would, with perfect logic, come out on exactly the opposite side of a question. She was fifty-eight years old when my children began to assert their authority when watching TV. I told mother that I only was going to let them watch programs I deemed suitable, assuming she would agree.

She was horrified. That I would be a censor was against every principle with which she had reared me. I was severely chastened. After long discussion, we settled on letting the children choose which one-hour period (not to be accumulated) they would watch each day. Mother breathed a sigh of relief. I was amazed at her ardor about the issue.

She was a very busy college student for a good part of my childhood. Despite teaching most of her life, she had not finished her degree and was always working on it. She finally got it when I was eighteen. We graduated together, I from high school and she from college. When I went to college, she went on for her master's degree in geography. She would have gone on for a PhD. but the university Dad was teaching in would not let her into the PhD program since the university would not hire her. There was a rule against nepotism, at least for wives, and the department concluded that she would not be able to use her degree, and therefore, the space should go to someone less deserving who could use the degree.

Mother was furious. My grandmother had finished only the eighth grade because her wealthy farmer father thought that a girl's place was helping her mother with the chores. All of her brothers went to high school, but she, the best student among them, had to stay at home. My grandmother imbued every one of her six children with a thirst for knowledge and swore that they would all get an education. They did. Among her six children there were one nursing degree, three master's degrees in education, and two doctorates.

I glanced at Dad whom I'm sure had eaten his sandwich without tasting it. I handed him a banana, and his twenty-ounce bottle of water. He still looked glum.

"You know, Dad," I said, "a lot of people see themselves as damaged. They don't see the well side; only the sick side. It's the old story about the glass. Is it half full or half empty?" I tried to console him. "You are eighty percent there. It's just that you miss your old self. You remember how you could think before your stroke. You still think a lot better than most people who've never had a stroke. Why don't you look at it that way?"

I tried to cheer him up with that excellent piece of logic. I didn't work. Emotions seldom respond to logical thoughts.

"I have never had my inability to think measured before. I think I would rather not know how damaged my brain actually is," he concluded.

We headed back to our little Pontiac Sunfire for the short drive to the place we were to get the MRI. It was in a strip mall full of other medical offices. I tried to park in the shade. Dad shuffled into the office, and again, I filled out forms. After twenty minutes we were called into the back.

Rachel, our technician, readied the flat bed where Dad was to lie down and position his head. "How long is this going to take?" I asked.

"About thirty minutes." Rachel said. "If you want to go into the room with him you'll have to take off your watch. This machine stops watches on a regular basis." I removed Dad's watch and glasses. He used to say that he couldn't hear with his glasses off, and then wait for the delayed reaction to his joke.

"I need to go to the bathroom first," Dad said. Rachel pointed to the door.

"May I stay out here with you?" I asked.

"Of course," she said.

Dad emerged from the washroom and Rachel took him into the MRI room. The machine was in the center of the dull beige chamber. It had two matching ten-foot discs, each three feet thick, with a space between them. A long flat bed containing the patient slid into the space. Rachel sat Dad down on the bed and gently turned him so that he was lying on his back with his head in a brace. She propped his knees up with a cushion. Then she slid him under the top disc.

"Are you claustrophobic?" she asked.

"No." Cheerful music was playing. Dad began to hum.

"You must stay absolutely still when we run this machine. Can you do that?"

"No singing?" Dad asked. He turned on all his charm when he was with a pretty girl. I loved watching him.

"No singing," commanded Rachel.

"I could use a nap. Can I go to sleep?"

"Of course. Ready?"

"Yes."

We left the room and closed the door. Next to the MRI room was a room with a big window looking in on the machine, with my Dad inserted into it like a giant lollipop stick. Rachel sat at a desk with a computer screen and lots of buttons and knobs. I sat in a rattan chair with a soft cushion on the seat.

In a few minutes, the computer screen displayed a perfect profile of my father's head. However, it was cut, top to bottom right through the center. I could see half of his brain, his spine with each vertebra, his eye sockets, nose, and jaw. I could even see the layer of fat that lay under his skin at the back of his neck. All of it was as crisp and clear as a black and white photograph.

"Unbelievable!" I said "This is absolutely unbelievable technology! I can see the inside of his head in the middle of his skull. How can they do that?"

"It is pretty amazing." Rachel said. The machine took a long time to finish taking the necessary pictures. But I didn't mind. The fact that humans had invented a machine that could take a picture of the inside of a head without ever disturbing flesh and bones needed some time to ponder.

Rachel stopped the machine and opened the door to the MRI room. She slid Dad out of the machine and put his head into a different head brace.

"Dad, you would not believe what I just saw. I saw the middle of your brain, and your spine and everything."

"Any secrets in there I don't know about?" he teased.

"Lie still again." Rachel pushed him back inside the slit between the two discs.

The second sets of pictures were ear-to-ear cross sections of his brain. She put several different parts of his brain on the screen at the same time. "See that dark spot on the bottom of his brain?" She pointed to a small black triangle. "That's the stroke. I don't usually see them so far down on the bottom."

The final set of pictures was of the left carotid artery that Debbie had not been able to see on the ultrasound. It was as clear as a drawing by Leonardo da Vinci. I could even see one little section that had narrowed to half the size of the rest of the artery.

"It's not blocked," I said.

Rachel twirled a few dials and punched some keys. "We will send the pictures to a radiologist to read." She stood up and looked at Dad through the window. "That's it. You're done." She opened the door of Dad's room and pulled his head out of the narrow hole. "Be careful when you get up," she cautioned him as she removed the head brace. "You might be a little dizzy."

"I've known about these machines," I said. "I've read about them in magazines, but nothing I read prepared me for what I actually saw on the screen. Dad, I could see the place you had the stroke. I could see your arteries, even the place where your carotid artery narrows."

"Did I look smart?" he asked.

"Not as smart as you used to," I countered.

"That's why I'm here, to get to be as smart as I used to be."

"Why do you need to be as smart as you used to be?" I knowingly fell into his trap as I slipped his glasses back on his head.

"So I can outsmart you," he chuckled. "Get me my cane and my watch, will you please?"

"They're right here." I handed them to him. "Bye, Rachel," I called as we left. I felt as if I knew her intimately because we had shared this amazing experience of seeing my father's mind. It occurred to me that she might now know his mind better than I did.

"That's it Dad. We are done for the day. How about going out to dinner? It's five o'clock. I'm tired. I bet you are, too."

"I'm exhausted." Dad closed his eyes as soon as he got in the car.

"We had a lot of stress today, Dad. We expected everything to go well and then we hit a few rough spots. I know you were disappointed when we couldn't see the doctor this morning. Then when we got to the psychologist's office and the appointment was at the wrong time, it was another hassle."

"These things happen."

"Yeah, but...," I began.

"Second cousin to a rabbit, the yeahbut." He told the old family joke, but without a smile.

"When things don't happen the way they are supposed to it makes me feel bad because I am the one who got you into this situation. If things don't work out, it's my fault for bringing you here." My own built-up tension poured out in a self-indulgent though truthful confession.

"The only way you could blame yourself would be if you hadn't brought me here. If I had missed this opportunity it would've been a tragedy. We just had a slow day. We have two-and-a-half more weeks here. We'll be fine." But his voice sounded flat and weary.

We drove north along the bay until we came to the Sea Sea Rider Restaurant. Dad struggled out of the car and slammed the door behind him. He hobbled to a chair by the window and propped his cane against the wall.

The waitress appeared. "Can I get you a drink?"

"Yes," Dad said at once.

"No," I said at the same time. "Dad, you are not supposed to drink."

"I'm not taking those pills yet. This may be my last drink and I'm going to have it. I'll have a martini with two olives," he said to the waitress.

"Yes sir," she said. I ordered white wine.

"You're going to go out in style," I said, smiling at his assertion of his will.

"If I can't drink anymore, I really want to enjoy this one."

The waitress brought our drinks and Dad raised his in a toast. As we clinked glasses, I said," Good luck, Dad. I hope this works."

"Maybe it will," he said, tentatively. "Maybe it will."

12

Partners

Friday, October 6

Day Four, Medication Day One

Dad and I dressed in black. He looked like Johnny Cash. I looked like Elvira. We were partners in an adventure. When we arrived at the Institute at eleven-thirty, the outer waiting room was empty. Where the day before every seat had been taken and the room crowded with people in wheelchairs, today, no one was rushing around. Patients had gotten early appointments so they could go home for the weekend.

In the main waiting room there was a lone woman in a wheelchair. She hardly looked human. Her body was flat, like a board stuck on top of the chair. Pink slipper socks encased her feet, although they looked like mittens on the end of spastic sticks. Her ankles were arched forward and her toes were pointed straight down. Her arms were stiffly aligned with her rigid body. She had no eyes, just slits closed tight. Her mouth was wide open and her tongue protruded. She did not move. She was there with a hired nurse, who came out of a back room and touched her gently on her shoulder before wheeling her to the front door. Summer ran to hold it open. There were people who were much worse than my father. We were lucky.

We were directed immediately into the office where we had waited the day before. I noticed all the model sailboats scattered around the room, an unframed canvas, a framed baby picture, and empty cardboard boxes under the credenza. It had the look of an alpha company that is expanding so rapidly it hasn't had time to create an image with décor. Sharon took Dad's blood pressure; it was up to 149/83. That was impressive for a man who earlier in the week had hit 98/60.

I took off Dad's shoes and socks again. Within minutes, a man in a white coat entered and sat down at the desk.

"This is Dr. Webber," Sharon said as she left.

Dr. Webber had a red face and was partially bald with a fringe of short white hair. His clear blue eyes were tentative, almost shy. I thought if he were a student in my class he would never raise his hand or volunteer, but he would always know the right answer if I called on him.

"My name is Robin Robinson and this is my father, Dr. Robinson." I used the title my father had worked so hard to earn so that the doctor would realize that my father was an important and intelligent person, not just another stroke victim. Not a person identified by his infirmity, but a person who was loved and respected by his family. Not to be dismissed, but to be honored. I had been in many doctors' offices. I was not going to be intimidated. Maybe it was a reaction to the doctor having been too busy to see us the day before. More likely, it was a reaction to years of doctors who were dismissive and uninterested in my problems. I was wary.

"What did you get your degree in?" Dr. Webber asked. He spoke quietly and Dad strained to hear him.

"Educational psychology," Dad said.

"You must have had fun in Dr. Gimon's office."

"Yesterday's examination was a strange experience," Dad admitted. "I was taking the examination Weschler Test that I had administered for years.

"I used to be his guinea pig as he demonstrated to his classes the proper way to administer the test. Even I know the test by heart," I said. "Dad, Dr. Webber is from Minnesota," I said using a fact that I had picked up from the blue binder information, which of course I have read cover to cover.

"Where in Minnesota?" Dad asked.

"Minneapolis."

"Dad used to teach in St. Cloud, at the teacher's college." There was a pause as he read Dad's file. "What is your specialty? The blue book says you are certified but doesn't tell in what."

"Geriatric medicine. I worked in a lot of retirement homes there." He began asking questions about Dad's stroke. I produced the few medical records that we'd been able to get from his last surgery, and the packet of records from his stroke that Lia had got from County Hospital.

"Dr. Robinson, your MRI came in this morning. I can see where the stroke occurred. Do you know what caused the stroke?" Dr. Webber asked.

"I always wanted to know," Dad said.

"Here it is," the doctor said, reading the medical records. An ischemic stroke. A blood vessel was blocked by a thrombus, a clot. We don't know why that happens. It was not caused by bleeding from a vein."

"Is that what causes all of my pain?"

"Probably. It's thalamic pain, brain-originated pain."

"If I could get rid of the pain…"

"He takes Ibuprofen for it," I added.

"Does it help?"

"Not much. It takes the edge off it. Maybe ten percent. I'm in pain all the time, except when I sleep. That's why I sleep so much, to escape the pain."

Doctor Webber began asking questions about Dad's medical history, filling out more forms. Then he did some tests on his reactions and his ability to move the side of his body affected by the stroke. I had to take off Dad's shoes and socks.

"We are going to start you on medications today," he said.

I drew a quick breath. I was surprised that he was going to begin so soon. But I was excited, as well. This was really the beginning. This was the day we might see changes. Maybe there would be changes in the first hour, or even in the first five minutes.

"Sharon will give you a shot of magnesium," Dr. Webber said. "It absorbs faster as a shot. You will also take 500 milligrams of magnesium daily. Ask the pharmacist to show you the magnesium gluconate, but you can buy it over the counter. Second, you will use nitroglycerin cream. Rub this much," he indicated a small amount, "on the skin of your affected arm and leg four times a day. Finally, take Lipitor twice a day. This drug is used predominately for lowering cholesterol."

"I don't have high cholesterol," Dad said.

"It is also a vessel dilator. We have had great success using it. These doses are specific to you, Dr. Robinson. We will be adjusting them almost daily." He handed Dad two sheets of paper. "The top sheet is a prescription. The second sheet tells you when to take the medications."

The second page looked like this:

Nitroglycerin Cream – 1-1-1-1
Lipitor – 1-0-1-0
Magnesium – 1-1-1-1
64 ounces of water

The doctor explained that the numbers indicated the medications that were to be taken at breakfast-lunch-dinner-bedtime. Dad began to rise. "Stay here for your magnesium shot," Dr. Webber said. "It's been a pleasure meeting you, Dr. Robinson."

He was cheerful and thorough and had listened to us carefully. Altogether, it was a pleasant experience, despite my apprehensions. I was proud that he had addressed my father with respect, as 'Doctor.' "Thank you, Doctor Weber," I said.

And so we had it!

We had the prescription for the medicines, the precious stuff. I felt as though I had just discovered the Fountain of Youth and sneaked a long drink behind some Florida Seminole's back.

Still, in a corner of my mind, I thought, "What if this entire operation is a scam? It could be a set-up, like an elaborate episode of 'Mission Impossible.' All of the people in the waiting room could be hired actors and this whole place could be phony. It all could be a ruse to take our $5,000."

I realized that I was being melodramatic. I knelt down to put Dad's socks on once more. Be realistic, Robin, I told myself. Putting on another adult's socks was a lesson in realism.

Sharon came in with the shot. "This is going to hurt," she warned.

"Put it in the arm that has no feeling," I said.

"You should take that prescription to the Highland Pharmacy. They are accustomed to our patients and understand what we are doing. Other places call and give us a hard time. Pharmacists want to substitute medications and that is not acceptable. It takes a lot of time to explain that to them." Sharon handed us the address and directions to the pharmacy.

A tingle ran though my body, the kind of tingle I felt before I left to meet Steve in Hawaii on our first trip together, or when I got the five-year $60,000 a year CAPE arts integration grant for Lincoln Park High School. Dad was beginning therapy today.

"How do you feel, Dad? Are you excited?"

"A little pessimistic," he said. "This may not work."

"Well, I'm excited! It's the beginning. Maybe something will happen right away."

"And maybe it won't," he said. "I don't want to get my hopes up."

The pharmacy bill was $398.76. Now I understood why there was a page in the blue folder about ordering drugs from Canadian or Mexican pharmacies. Luckily for Dad, his insurance policy covered most of it and we were left with a bill for $83. This one went on the Discover card. Visa had already had quite a workout with the doctor, the educational psychologist, and the physical therapist.

He started medications as soon as we got back to the motel.

13
Changes
Saturday, October 7
Day Five, Medication Day Two

"I feel better," Dad said, over his raisin bran the next morning. "I don't know, maybe I'm fooling myself, but if I am to heck with it. It's good. I feel better."

"How do you feel better?" I asked.

"I am thinking better. You can't make a silk purse out of a sow's ear, but these doctors are trying." He paused a minute. "Do you realize that I just remembered a proverb? That's something new."

"Anything else?" I asked.

"I can walk better. And my arm hurts less."

Outside the window a lizard scampered over a cement-block fence and down into a cactus plant. Another one sat in the sun, its head and tail up in the air in expectation, just as we waited, alert and expectant, for changes in Dad. Suddenly the lizard blew up a huge orange air sack under his chin. His body jerked up and down as he drew attention to his beauty, with his explosion of orange. It was a demonstration of change, proof that change was possible. All we had to do was wait and watch.

Dad insisted on closing his own door when we went to the car, even though he had to do it with his bad right hand. He got hold of the door in two attempts. That was faster than before. At least I thought it might be faster. Maybe I was wrong.

We had a free day to do grocery shopping and to return to Wal-Mart to exchange the way-too-big clothes that I had bought for Dad on our first trip there. I had measured his waist at forty-seven inches. When we got home and he tried on the shorts, they were huge. I'd measured wrong or he must have lost weight. I had been making him eat very nutritiously. I bought black pants and blue, green, and plaid shorts in size forty-four. That way I wouldn't have to do laundry every day. He would have plenty of shorts to wear.

Dad never shopped for himself. If mother didn't buy it for him, he didn't have it. It had been six years since she'd been well enough to go shopping for him. Since that time my sister had been in charge. She hated shopping as much as Dad did, so he'd looked a little scruffy the past few years.

My father is a good-looking man. His skin was unwrinkled, even at eighty-two. He'd smoked most of his life and I distinctly remember that his skin used to be an ashen gray. After the stroke, he quit smoking. That had been eight years ago and now his skin was pink and healthy. His dusky blue eyes and smiling face made people feel at ease.

That evening, Mark, the young fisherman who was staying in the next room at the motel, knocked on our door. "Do you want me to get some shrimp tomorrow morning? I'll go at six and see if I can find some big ones. That's when the boats come in."

"Fresh shrimp! Never frozen? Absolutely!'

"I'm going to barbecue." He pointed to a big brick grill.

"May we join you?"

"Sure."

14
Whom Can We Tell?
Sunday, October 8
Day Six, Medication Day Three

The next afternoon we feasted on skewered shrimp, tomatoes, onions, and green peppers over rice. It was great to eat something that was not my cooking. Having a conversation with someone other than Dad was a novelty and felt good, too. Dad's wit was running full throttle. He made joke after joke and kept us laughing. I hadn't seen him like that since before the stroke.

After lunch, we walked around the swimming pool and out to the fishing dock, exercising Dad's legs a bit. "I think my ankle works a little better," he said.

"You think? Does it or doesn't it?"

"I don't know. I can't really tell. I'm probably imagining it." He plodded on around the pool. "I think my toes are bending, too. There is this funny feeling in the heel of my foot. Like a tingle."

"I'm supposed to keep track of just that kind of thing," I said. "I'll write it down as soon as we get inside." I pulled out the pages on which we had painstakingly checked off Dad's symptoms. On the bottom I wrote the date and "thinks his ankle and toes are bending, tingly feeling in heel-right side." Dad had been on medications for two days.

There was an ever-so-slight change, just what we'd been told to look for, the beginning of greater changes to come.

In the back of my mind, like a tune that kept playing, was a call I'd been meaning to make to old friends of mine from Chicago. They had retired and moved to Bradenton, about an hour's drive south of Clearwater. Sixteen years before, their daughter, Heather, was driving home from a wedding rehearsal when her car was hit by first one truck and then another. Heather had been an actress and a college student, and one of the most cheerful and optimistic people on earth. After the accident she was paralyzed. She could not move voluntarily. She could not hold her head up. She could not even swallow. But she could look at you with a twinkle in her eyes. She could watch the soaps on TV. She could flirt with her favorite people, mostly men.

When the accident happened, Heather's parents, Brooks and Dorothy, had been working for a non-profit organization, counseling village developments in Africa. They'd come home immediately, and had been taking care of Heather ever since. They'd had help from a series of hired nurses, but Heather had to be turned every two hours, and washed, and fed, and her diaper changed. Her parents also felt it necessary to keep her stimulated with trips to the beach and daily sessions in the swimming pool. I admired them enormously for their courage, patience, and the love they lavished on their daughter.

I thought that the Institute might be able to help Heather, if I could only get them to take her there. Dr. Hammesfahr had treated many accident victims with closed head injuries. He'd been given a commendation from the Vietnam's Veteran's Association for his work with the closed head injuries of institutionalized veterans. I had sent Brooks and Dorothy some information about the Institute but hadn't discussed it with them yet.

Dorothy answered the phone. "Let's get together while Dad and I are down here," I said.

"We are having problems getting an afternoon nurse right now. We can't really get away. Do you think you could come down here?"

"Sure."

"Next weekend we have guests. How about the weekend after that? Come for lunch."

"Great." I got the directions for the drive to their home. "Did you get the information that I sent you from Dr. Hammesfahr's office?"

"Yes, but we haven't looked at it yet."

"Look at it, Dorothy. And pull up that web site, HNI-Online.com. I really think it could help Heather."

"We are worried that if she gets better she will lose her lovely disposition. She might be much harder to care for than before."

I hadn't thought of that problem.

15

To Feel Again

Monday, October 9

Day Seven, Medication Day Four

A cold front moved through Clearwater during the night and we awoke shivering in 58-degree weather. The sky was cloudy and depressing. I closed all the windows to try to keep what heat we had in the rooms. "We have Chicago weather this morning. This is the way it is all winter in Chicago. Cloudy and cold."

"I'm not taking a shower this morning," Dad said, as I took his blood pressure. It was 130/80. Right where it was supposed to be to begin new medications, a little high.

"Oh yes you are," I told him, sniffing his smelly body. "Did you change your underwear?"

"Okay, but let me wait until it's a little warmer."

I made his breakfast and prepared his medications. Then I started a pot of hot coffee to warm him up. "Here's your water." I handed him a twenty-ounce bottle.

"I'm not going to drink it today," Dad protested. "It makes me pee all the time."

"Oh yes you are. Do you want this medicine to work or not? How do you feel this morning?"

"Just the same. No difference."

"You won't complete the third full day of your medication until supper. You have seven more days to go before the time most people feel something. Don't lose heart now. You're just beginning."

Suddenly, the sun broke through the clouds and bathed the canal beside our rooms in light. I felt better immediately. Fie on my dermatologist. I love the sun.

The phone rang. It was Lia calling to give me her vacation address. She was cheerful and happy to be off for a week and headed north, to cold Wisconsin. "I like it that way," she said. "I'd rather be cold than hot."

I told her about the MRI.

"You should read 'Timeline,'" she said. "It's about time travel. They find a man whose blood vessels don't line up. It looks as though he was beamed down but there was a glitch in the process, so scientists study his body with an MRI. It's quantum physics," she added. "An MRI is our first practical use for quantum physics."

I promised to get it the next time I went shopping.

I asked her about Dad's pharmacy in Rock Island. She assured me that there was a pharmacy two blocks away from the Fort Armstrong that delivered prescriptions. Dad talked to her for a few minutes about his finances.

"She said she'll call back when she gets home," he told me.

It felt good to have my sister back on my side. We got in the car and put on a CD. Ella Fitzgerald was singing and Dad sang along with her.

"From this moment on,
You and I dear,
We'll be flying high dear,
From this moment on."

His whole mood had changed. Music is amazing.

When we get to the Institute, Angela was in the waiting room. "Do you live here?" I teased. "Every time we come to this office you are sitting in that chair."

"I can't get my blood pressure to stabilize. First it's too high and then it's too low. I sit here all day every day.

Today is so cold." She pulled the collar of her of her sweater up around her neck with her good hand.

"When are you going home?" I asked.

"I'm flying back to Pensacola tomorrow. This is my last day." A nurse brought Angela some lunch. "I even eat here. They order out for me."

"You look so pretty today. Do you put on your lipstick with your left hand?"

"Yes," she said.

"You're good at it."

"Thanks," she said, and laughed a little.

Debbie, the technician, took us into a side living room. "Let me get another blood pressure from you," she said, as she rolled up Dad's sleeve.

"I don't have any more if it," he protested lightly. "You took it all yesterday."

It was 165/84. Dr. Webber arrived and looked at the numbers. "Good," he said. "Your blood pressure is high enough to begin Accupril, another vessel dilator."

"Why is it so high?" I asked.

"Did you eat breakfast?"

"Yes."

"Did you take your medications?"

"Yes."

"Did you drink your sixty-four ounces of water?"

"Yes."

That is probably why it went up. Drinking water affects the pressure in your blood vessels," the doctor explained.

"It also makes me pee all the time," Dad countered.

"Your bladder will eventually get used to it and you won't have so much trouble."

"Why do I sleep all the time? Is that related to my blood pressure?"

"Poor circulation probably causes your tiredness. As the blood vessels dilate your energy level will increase. We are aiming for a target blood pressure from 120/70 to 140/70." He handed us a new form that said Accupril (5mg) 1-1-1-1. "Did you get this medicine last week with your other prescriptions?"

"Yes, we did."

"Start it with lunch today. Any other questions?"

"No."

"See you tomorrow. Drink your water." He left the room and we started for the car. Dad began to sing.

"The stars at night,
Are big and bright,
Deep in the heart of Texas.
Reminds me of
The one I love,
Deep in the heart of Texas."

That was a hopeful song for the day. I suddenly noticed that dad was singing more often this week. As we left the building, a nurse wheeled out the patient who'd been perfectly rigid the day before. She was sitting up in her wheelchair. Her ankles were no longer arched and her feet were on the footrests. Her eyes were open, but vacant, and her mouth was closed.

"Look, Dad," I said. "That's the woman we saw yesterday who was like a board in her chair. She's sitting up today. That's remarkable!" Although it was rude, we both stopped and stared at her a moment before we got into the car. Her glazed eyes still saw nothing but her own inner confusion. Ours saw hope.

At six we took our nightly walk around the motel swimming pool. The wind was strong and cold. It was low tide and hundreds of birds were feeding in the sea grass. We stopped and watched the white and blue herons and the pelicans. Little egrets picked at the oysters along the shoreline. The pelicans dove into the water and held their position until they straightened out their catches in their necks and swallowed them. They were so focused on what they were doing, it was beautiful. I could have watched for hours, but it was cold, so we walked on.

"Robin, my knee is really bending." Dad looked down at his leg.

"Didn't it bend before?" I asked.

"No. I used to walk like this." He demonstrated a stiff-kneed gait. "Now look. I can bend it when I walk."

"Does it still hurt?"

"Yes, but I didn't take my Ibuprofen at lunch today."

"Maybe the pain is subsiding."

"Not right now, it's not. But it is a different kind of pain. My leg feels all tingly. Like it was asleep. I can feel my toe bend inside my shoe and that funny feeling I had yesterday in my heel is gone. Maybe I'm fooling myself, but I hope not." He paused to shift his weight to his good leg before starting down a small step. We crossed the parking lot. "My arm is swinging, too. It's not stiff."

"Whoa!" That was really something. His knee was bending. His arm was swinging at his side. I could see these differences. "I'll write this down as soon as we get inside, next to the lines I wrote last night. It will be great news for the doctors tomorrow."

"I feel like I have a face again, too." Dad said. "I can feel my right side tingle." He rubbed his face. "Yes, I can feel it."

He had been on medication only four days.

I wished we had a bottle of wine in the room to celebrate. I vowed to buy one the next day. Then I remembered that Dad could not drink wine. We would have to toast with our water bottles.

When we got inside I arranged the magnetic letters that I bought at the Dollar Store to say I LOVE U on the refrigerator.

After dinner, as I was getting involved in a copy of "Timeline," Dad called to me, "Robin, come here a minute. Do I have a fever?"

"Let me feel your head." I had raised three children and I knew when one of them was faking a fever. I felt his head. He was perspiring, but he had no fever. "I think you're having a hot flash," I said. "Let's wait a half an hour and see if you're still hot."

When I checked later, he had no symptoms. I noted the incident in his journal.

16
Sugar Daddy
Tuesday, October 10
Day Eight, Medication Day Five

I awoke just after eight. The place was quiet and I couldn't hear the TV. Dad always got up early and turned it on. It usually woke me up. I listened intently as I looked out the window. The sky had a few white clouds against the blue. There was a small thrush perched on a high wire, taking a bath. I wondered if it was still cold. Why wasn't my father up? What if something had happened during the night? What if his blood pressure got very low and he couldn't get up? I climbed out of bed and turned the corner to the kitchen.

There he was. The TV was on, but very low. "How you doing?" I asked, as I moved to the back of his chair and kissed him behind his ear.

"I am totally disoriented. Where are we? What are we doing here?" he looked bewildered. "I have no idea where we are or why we are here."

I sat down on the couch. "Where do you live?" I asked.

"I don't know."

"What time of year is it?"

He shook his head.

"What month is it?"

He was silent.

"What is the date? The year?"

Still no answer.

"What happened to me?" he asked.

"I don't know." I was frightened. This behavior was not usual. I had never seen him so disoriented. I started putting the dishes from the drying rack back in the cabinets. The first thing I do when I'm disturbed is to begin cleaning up, as though I can bring about a return to normalcy by performing mundane tasks. I fixed Dad's raisin bran and orange juice. "Come and eat breakfast, Dad. Turn off the television. Maybe you'll feel better after you eat."

"I think we're in Florida," he guessed, as he moved to the kitchen table.

I handed him his water bottle. "Drink some," I said.

He ate breakfast while I got out the nitroglycerin cream and his pills for the morning dose.

"Why are we here?" he asked again.

I relented. "You are here to see if the doctors can reverse the symptoms of your stroke and make you walk well again."

"Oh, yes." He ate quietly.

A few minutes later he said, "Why are we here?"

"Dad, I just told you. Don't you remember?"

"No."

I filled out the forms we had to turn in each day that identified what medications he had taken in the last twenty-four hours. He looked on with interest. Then he took his pills and I put the nitro cream on his arm.

He took another drink of orange juice. "I think I remember. We are going to take the car and go to Druid Street and see that doctor."

"That's right."

"It's coming back to me now. We go into a house and I sit across a bench from him."

"Table. That's right," I said.

"He's trying to find something out."

"Right. Do you know what?"

"No."

Dad was looking at the flowers I'd bought to make the motel room a little less impersonal. "Those are beautiful peonies," he said. "No, not peonies, what are they? Carnations. They're carnations."

"Exactly." I began to clear off the breakfast dishes.

"I can remember now. Did I have another stroke?"

"I don't think so. If you had you wouldn't be able to remember things now."

"I remembered where I was when I got up and got dressed. It was just when I was watching TV that I couldn't remember anything. I haven't had a spell like that before, not that I know of."

"What time of year is it?"

"Fall."

"What month?"

"October."

"You didn't know that ten minutes ago. You did click your fingers across the tabletop. Excellent tapping.

"My leg and arm feel worse."

"When you went to bed last night you said they felt pretty good."

"I can think better, but I still can't walk. I can't move my arm," he sighed. "I want everything to happen BANG! and be fixed."

"I know you're frustrated, but improving is a process, little by little. We'll ask the doctor about your disorientation when we get there this morning. Let's go right away." I wouldn't say so, but I was concerned that he might have had a mini stroke. I needed to know for sure.

The parking lot was full to overflowing with a line waiting to get in when we arrived. We had to wait for someone to leave before we could park. Inside we found a place to sit, but there was a long list of people ahead of us who had not been called into the doctors' offices yet.

The waiting room was always a nice place to be because there were so many friendly people there. We introduced ourselves. A man and his wife across the room, Neil and Jean, turned out to be from Chicago.

"How did you find out about this place?" I asked.

"A friend at Northwestern University recommended it," Neil said. "Then my daughter found brochures for it at the hospital where she's doing her internship. Last week I couldn't talk. Now I can. Isn't that something!"

He was in a wheelchair. His arm and leg were in braces. He was a strong-looking man, compact and well-built. His brown hair was nicely trimmed and he looked as though he'd had a manicure.

"This is our second week here," he said. "Hey, there's my angel." Neil pointed to Dr. Uzo, a tall black woman, as she hurried by.

She wore big gold earrings and a bright print shirt under her doctor's coat. She didn't look like an ordinary angel, but she sure looked powerful.

"I have to go to the bathroom every hour," Neil continued unabashedly. "I can't even leave the house without wearing a diaper. I have a bladder problem."

"So do I," Dad said.

"Maybe this treatment will help," I said.

"I was really bad," Neil went on. "I couldn't talk."

"Now he can think again," his wife said, finally getting a word in edgewise. "We can actually have a conversation."

"I had the stroke in December," Neil said. His tongue sometimes slipped and inserted an extra syllable as he spoke. "I had a triple by-pass and a clot. They asked Jean if she wanted to pull the plug. Thank God she didn't. I wasn't sick a day in my life before that. Only God knows."

"And He ain't talking," finished Dad.

Obviously, Neil was enjoying his newfound speech. He had ten months of silence to make up for, and he was going at it full steam. "We're going to buy a condo here," he said. "We went to look at one yesterday. They are building it over on Clearwater Beach."

"Oh, I don't know," Jean said. "We will go and look at the plans. But he does understand finances again. That's a big relief."

"We're going to buy it. Get out of those cold winters." Neil was still talking when a patient named Ted interrupted.

"The first time we were out after my stroke and I had to go to the bathroom, Suzy took me," he said, indicating his wife. "We wheeled into the bathroom and I realized that there were all stalls and no urinals. It was the women's bathroom. I could see her through the crack in the stall door when she walked out and left me in there alone."

"I was going to stand by the door so that no women went in until he got out," Suzy said.

"She didn't understand the paranoia that goes with a stoke," Ted said." So the next time I made her take me to the men's room. I stood by the urinal and struggled to get my pants down. Then I had to hold on to the plumbing to steady myself. I couldn't aim with my bad hand so Suzy had to aim. So then she gets cute and starts spraying it all over when a guy comes in the door, stops dead, and just stares at the scene.

'Don't worry,' I shouted at him. 'She's new at this!' He turned and walked out of the bathroom. What else could I say without being demeaning to my caretaker, my wife?"

Everyone in the waiting room roared with laughter. They'd all had their own difficulties with basic human activities.

Soon Sharon came and ushered us into the area reserved for appointments. There were two such stations in the room, with a curtain between them. Three easy chairs formed a small group in each area, with a bedside table where Sharon placed Dad's records. She was taking Dad's blood pressure as Neil's angel, Dr. Uzo, came by in her Dr. Scholl's sandals. "Hi, Robin. Kiss, kiss," she said, and gave Dad a hug.

"Now you can blame Dr. Uzo for your high blood pressure," Sharon teased. All this excitement must have revved Dad up because by the time they took his blood pressure it had gone to 137/75. Perfect.

Little bits of conversation floated in from other rooms.

"Could I have a smaller number of pills? I don't have enough money for all of them."

"Am I doing magnesium drips today?"

"I didn't use my patch. I didn't have anymore patches."

"Your blood pressure is okay today."

Dr. Uzo read Dad's charts. We described the morning's disorientation.

"Did you give him something to eat?" she asked me.

"Yes, orange juice and raisin bran."

"Good, lots of sugar. That's probably what helped him. I think he might have had low blood sugar. Do you usually eat more sweets?"

"I usually eat Milky Way candy bars before I go to bed," Dad confessed.

"I have kept him on a very healthy diet," I said. "No candy."

"You might give him something sweet before bedtime. No chocolate though. I'm going to give you an order for a blood sugar test early tomorrow morning. Do not eat or drink before you go. It will say diabetes on the order. Don't pay any attention to that. I just need a blood sugar test." She handed us the order. "Have you noticed any other changes?"

"Yes," Dad said. "I can bend my knee. I used to walk with it stiff. Now I can bend it when I take a step. It feels odd. I'm not used to it."

"That's good," Dr. Uzo said. "Even a little progress is good, and that is where you will improve first." She wrote on the chart. "I'd like to increase your Accupril to three pills in the evening." She wrote out an order: 1-1-1-3. These shorthand directions for dosage were very clear and easy to follow. Dad took one pill at breakfast, one at lunch, and one at dinner. Before he went to bed he took three. "You're doing great to see changes already," the doctor said. "How long have you been taking medicine?"

"I don't know. Robin?"

I counted the days. "Since Friday afternoon, four and a half days."

"Remarkable," she smiled. "You just keep it up. Are you going to the education meeting this afternoon?"

"Are we?" Dad asked.

"You bet your booties," I said. "It starts at two-thirty. We'll be there."

We returned to the motel for lunch before the meeting. Dad rearranged the magnetic letters on the refrigerator to say YU LOVE I. We only had one of each letter so all of our writing looked dyslectic, but we didn't care. Spelling was not on our list of important things, and creative spelling was fun.

At the meeting, Diane Hartley, the physical therapist, spoke first. "How many of you administer shots of magnesium?" she began. About a third of the audience raised their hands. "Let me give you some hints about how to do it." She went into a detailed explanation about how to use and store and warm the magnesium. I crept over to the food table and got two cookies and two bottles of water.

"Now I want to talk about new return," Diane said. "How many of you have new return?"

"What's that?" someone asked.

"Muscles that start working again after having been tensed for a long time." Hands shot up all over. "Good. That's what I expected. I'm going to go around the room to ask you about what movement has returned. Tell me everything that's happened. The smallest change is major. It indicates where the brain is healing itself."

We were first. "Can you do anything about the pain in my arm?" asked Dad.

"Yes," Diane said. "Positively." Enthusiasm exuded from her bouncy body. "When I was in pain from a car accident injury this is what I did. Soak your arm in Epsom salts. It's pure magnesium. It will help relieve the pain. Put two cups in a dishpan, add hot water to dissolve it, and then add some cold water to cool it down. Do it daily or whenever it hurts."

"My hand is beginning to loosen up," Dad said. "Should I exercise it with a squeeze ball?"

"Remember that your muscles are working after a long time of being tense. You have to notice what happens in the healing process." She picked up another patient's hands. "See her loosen and move them. Take your fingers and stretch them backwards with the fingers of your other hand," she said to the woman. "Stretch out the muscles and tendons in your hands. Hold your arm in a different position. Put a little pressure on it and push it down. If you exercise it, it will improve faster. The lack of use of the muscle causes the ligaments to shrink. They must be pulled out again."

Diane went from table to table showing caregivers and patients how to move their newly reactivated muscles. "Don't overdo it. Frequently and gently is best. Take your thumb in your good hand and twist it in a circle like you are winding it up." She took a woman's hand and demonstrated. "See her fingers relax. This is a great trick and it works every time. Do this a lot. The best time to exercise is one hour after you've used the nitro ointment. That is when it's most effective."

"What about water exercise?" someone asked.

"Electric stimulation?"

"Shoulder problems?"

The questions and answers flew back and forth until they were finally exhausted, and Diane introduced Dr. Alan Gimon.

Dr. Gimon was another of the Institute's cheerful types. He wore an open collared shirt and talked with his hands. "You have to practice with the brain as well as with your other muscles. Don't let patients just sit there. Make them do mental gymnastics. Use the exercises that you did in the WISC test. List all the words you can think of that begin with the letter 'a' or 'f.' Develop a system that follows the alphabet; words that begin with 'ab,' then 'ac,' then 'ad.' Use different letters. Ask them about politics. People who have had strokes can still vote. Make them decide what they think about issues that are important to them, like Medicare and Social Security. Are there any questions?"

"What about aphasia?" one woman asked. "What is it and how does it work?"

"You can have expressive aphasia and not be able to talk, but still be able to understand things," Dr. Gimon said. "There is also an aphasia of the language that the patients hears. These are two different things. Is your husband...?"

"He can't talk," she interrupted, as her husband made a few sounds and raised his finger to point.

"But he might understand." Dr. Gimon looked directly at the portly man with the red face. "Nod your head if you can hear me."

The man began to speak in unintelligible syllables and pointed his finger off to the left.

"If you can understand me, nod your head," the doctor repeated forcefully.

The man stopped pointing and mumbling. His head bobbed up and down.

"Is this your wife?"

"The man nodded.

"She must be a good wife if you admit it."

Everyone in the room laughed and the man smiled. "You see, he does understand. He has expressive aphasia, not receptive aphasia. Talk to him and make him answer you. Keep his mind stimulated with your questions."

A patient at our table stood and walked towards the bathroom. Sharon, the nurse, was right there to help her.

"She couldn't walk when we came here three months ago," her husband confided to Dad. "Look at her go now." He was as proud as if he had done it himself.

Dr. Uzo arrived next. She had changed out of her Dr. Scholl's sandals and into high-heeled fuchsia pumps. She hooked up the mike and began. "I don't want you to start comparing the medications that you are taking to those that other people are taking. Each patient is unique. Each patient's medications are unique. For those with low blood pressure, it will take three to six months longer for you to see progress than if you had higher blood pressure, but it will happen. It is just a bit slower process. We do not extrapolate from one course of treatment to another, and you should not compare yourself to other patients. We work for everyone to get better, but it is individual therapy."

I put my hand over my father's. He was holding his stroke-affected right hand down with his left so the right one didn't fly up in the air and float around. He had one of those low blood pressures that would be slow to heal.

"I want to talk to you a little about your eating," Dr. Uzo continued. "I want you to remember to keep drinking your water, sixty-four ounces every day. That helps metabolize the medicine. Space it out between eight in the morning and four in the afternoon, so you're not up all night going to the bathroom.

"If you must have a cup of coffee, have it in the morning and don't drink more than six ounces. More coffee could cause episodic ups and downs of your blood pressure.

Don't drink decaffeinated coffee. We don't know what is in that. "Do not use artificial sweeteners, some of those are vessel constrictors. No sodas. Drink juice or water instead. Read the labels. Everybody must like yogurt a lot because I keep getting questions on it so I went to the store today to check out the yogurt labels. Use low fat yogurt. No fat yogurt has artificial sweeteners in it.

"Alcohol causes problems with the medication so avoid it.

"Smoking causes *major* blood vessel constriction. And caregivers, if you smoke, it's not good enough to leave the room. Vascular constriction comes from the secondhand odor of the smoke on your clothes. You can't smoke outside and then come into the room. You have to take a shower and wash your clothes before you can see the patient. It is probably less trouble to quit smoking.

"You must control your weight so your heart pumps easier. Now is the time to go on a diet.

"The average adult should have only 300 milligrams of cholesterol a day. One egg is 271 milligrams. If you eat an egg, that egg contains all the cholesterol you can have that whole day. Eggbeaters are all right. We recommend no egg yolks, no bacon, and no sausages.

"You must make a whole lifestyle change. Drink your water. See your doctor at home once a month. When you come back in three months for a check-up, bring your blood pressures readings for the entire time that you have been away. We have changed the checkup to five days instead of three, because three days was not enough time to observe the effects of any changes in your medications." She finally paused long enough to allow someone to raise a hand.

"Why are there no scientific studies on this work by others?" asked man in a red shirt.

"It's not easy for a private physician to publish in a major medical journal," Dr. Uzo said. "His work is published on MedForum, which is a medical journal. Everything new now is published on the Internet." She pointed to another hand, but the question stuck with me. Why weren't there any articles published in other Medical journals? Why wasn't the whole world writing about this therapy? Why weren't other doctors flocking to the Institute to learn about it? I made a note to ask Dr. Hammesfahr.

"Do you use Accupril because it has a longer half life?" asked a caregiver in the middle of the room.

"We use Accupril because it works best," the doctor said.

"What should I do if my doctor is not cooperating?"

"Show him what has happened to you. Show him how you have improved. That should change his mind."

"Get a new doctor!" a woman shouted from the rear.

"We seem to have the most trouble with neurologists," Dr. Uzo said. "They do not understand the treatment and they do not think it will work. Cardiologists seem to understand and accept it more easily. You do need a doctor at home who cooperates. Most the of the GPs get on the bandwagon once they see your recovery."

She sounded as though she was winding down. Dad got up to go to the bathroom. Donna took over the meeting.

"We want to say hello to a few of our friends. Daniel, come up here. Daniel was here three months ago. He couldn't walk and his left arm and hand were frozen." Daniel walked up the podium without any noticeable limp. "Show us your hand." He raised his left hand up above his head. "Higher," Dr. Uzo demanded. He shot it straight up.

"I am so much better," he shouted in his English accent.

"Teva! Say hello to us," said Donna.

"Hello everyone," Teva responded. How are you?"

"Teva has been here two weeks," Donna said. "When she came she could not speak or even sit up in a chair. Now she can sit up by herself and can speak in short sentences."

From across the table, Teva's husband, Fred, could not resist leaning over and confiding, "My wife is giving me orders again. It comes and goes, but eventually she will talk all the time. Her legs are getting stronger and she can walk a lot better." Then the meeting broke up into individual discussions.

"Take the extra sandwiches home!" Donna shouted, handing out plastic take-home cases. "Don't leave these here. Eat the cookies."

As we left the Yacht Club, dad said, "Let's go out to dinner."

"You're on." I was delighted to be relieved of cooking duties for the night.

We got in the car and drove down Mandalay Avenue. Dad began to sing.

"On the road to Mandalay

Where the flying fishes play

And the dawn comes up like thunder out of China 'cross the bay."

"I have never heard you sing that song in my life. I thought I had heard every song that you knew. You're pulling new things out of your mind."

Dad and I were on another road, the long road to wellness. This "Road to Mandalay" was full of opportunity and risk, excitement and disappointment.

17

Gifts from God

Wednesday, October 11

Day Nine, Medication Day Six

At 7:45 AM there were ten people waiting outside the lab door for blood work. The parking lot was full. We stayed in the car and turned on the heat.

"I learned something last night when we watched that Florida Everglades program," Dad said.

"Something you're going to use, or is it like learning square roots?"

"It will keep my brain active, either way."

The radio blared, "The Dow Jones is down 8.4 percent so far this year."

"Better than thinking about the market," Dad said. "It's the pits."

By the time we noticed that the line was gone there were already twenty-one people in the waiting room. We were number twenty-two.

"They must have a special on blood letting today," Dad quipped.

It didn't take us long to get into the technician's room. There was one chair. "Do you sit in the chair or do I?" asked Dad, with a twinkle in his eye for the cute brunette who was going to pull several vials of blood from his arm.

"You get to sit. I stand." She tied off his arm and slipped the needle into the vein, all business. We were out of there in half an hour.

We headed back to the motel for a quick breakfast and shower, and were at the doctor's office by ten. I signed in and Dad made himself comfortable in a wing chair. I sat on the other side of the fireplace in another wing chair.

"Hi," I said to a couple across the room. "Where are you from?" It was hard not to be cheerful in that room, even while waiting for a doctor's appointment.

"We live in a small town outside Denver," the middle-aged woman said. "My name is Nancy and this is my husband, Dirk." Dirk was tanned and handsome. He didn't look like he'd had a stroke. But he didn't speak, either.

"I worked on a dude ranch in Colorado one summer," Dad said. "It was when I was a Music Major in college. I started out as a dishwasher. Right after I got there, the bandleader walked out. I told the owners that I could lead a band and sing. They tried me out and I was hired. I didn't have to wash any more dishes. When they found out that I spoke French I got to squire the German ambassador's wife around during the day. She was French."

"Where was the ranch?" asked Nancy.

"On Grand Lake," Dad said.

I was astounded! He had remembered the name of a place he had worked sixty-three years ago. His memory had been too impaired to do that just a few days earlier.

"I know where that is," Nancy said. "It's all national park now." She did all the talking. Dirk sat there, uninterested, or not comprehending, looking in the other direction.

"I visited it a few years ago," Dad said. "The dude ranch was still there, but it had been taken over by the government." This memory trick of his was getting to be very good.

We were sitting next to a young woman named Ellen, who was there with her mother. Ellen was beautiful, with clear pale skin and blonde hair that hung past her shoulders. Her hand was cinching up towards that classic stroke position over her heart.

"Do you tie your own shoes?" asked Nancy, pointing to Ellen's tennis shoes. Most of the patients used Velcro fasteners on their shoes.

"Yeah, you want me to show you?" Ellen pulled her laces apart and tied them with one hand, using her bad hand to secure a lace end and bracing her bad elbow between her knees. "I can tie only one loop, so I tuck the other end into my shoe."

"That is very inventive."

Ellen grinned broadly. "My bad hand is getting better since I came here last week. It's more relaxed and hangs down by my side sometimes. It makes me happy. If you have a limp you can always say, 'It's my ankle,' or something. If your arm is jammed against your chest everyone knows I'm a cripple."

I noticed that she changed pronouns from you to I in the middle of the sentence. Her psychological pain was probably as difficult for her as her physical problems. The big book bag by her side made her look like a college student. Young people do not want to stick out, to be different. I had spent thirty years teaching students who longed to be in cliques and clubs or known as Mod, or Goth, or Hip-Hop. Kids love to find things in common with each other. Not many had had a stroke.

Ellen stood to go. Her bad leg flung itself out in front of her and she careened onto it. She left the room limping profoundly.

And she was worried about her arm? I thought. She could hardly walk. My heart got a little crack in it.

Nancy and Dirk and Dad and I watched her mother take her into one of the offices. Dr. Raines rushed through. "Hi, everybody," he called in passing.

I turned back to Nancy. "How did you find out about this place?" I asked.

"It was a gift from God," she answered quietly.

"What do you mean?" I said.

"Dirk had his stroke ten years ago, but we still travel a lot. We have a twenty-four-foot motor home and were going to take it to Arizona for a month. We pulled into an RV camp that had a bingo game. During the game, a strange woman came up to me and asked if my husband had had a stroke.

'Yes,' I told her. Ten years ago.'

"'I have a phone number,' the woman said. 'I heard this doctor turns around strokes.' She held out a scrap of paper with the number scrawled on it.

"'Who is he?' I asked.

"'I don't know.'

"'Where is he located?'

"'I don't know that either. Look, do you want this or not?'

"'Sure,' I said. 'Thank you.' I never saw the woman again. When we got home, I called the number and the Institute sent out a packet of information, including the cost. I looked up the studies on the Internet. We yearned to come. But we didn't have the money. I work part time, but not enough to come up with $5,000. And then we found out there would be another $800 beyond that. And that Medicare didn't cover anything. I prayed to the Lord for a sign whether we were to do this or not."

"What happened?"

"Money started pouring in."

"From other people?"

"No, our money. We got a letter from AT&T. They wanted to buy back our Media One stock. Then we had a time-share in Vail that we had put on the market six years ago. It sold. We found out that we would need another $400 worth of prescriptions. A man who owed us money from a long time ago showed up and paid us off. That was enough of a sign. We had the money. We came."

"How long have you been here?"

"Just two days. We haven't even started the medication. How long have you been here?"

"Dad has been taking medication since last Friday."

"Do you see any change?" she asked, hopefully.

"Oh yes. We already see change."

Nancy took a deep breath. She looked at her husband. He was unable to reply, although he had understood. Now he was listening intently. I could see that he wanted to talk very much. I hoped he would.

"Everyone gets better." I echoed what appeared to be the mantra of the Institute.

A woman nearby was discussing shoes. "I had to buy two pair. One pair size thirteen and one pair size fourteen for his affected foot. His arch flattened out and his foot got bigger."

There were thousands of little things affected by a stroke that no one ever thinks about until confronted with them: how to tie a shoe, or put on a tie, or undo a pair of pants, or shake hands, or hold a cane and open a door. Even clapping was impossible with one hand.

We were called in for the ultrasound. Debbie got Dad in the chair and Sharon brought in his chart and took his blood pressure. It was 127/76. "You have perfect blood pressure," she said. "Are you drinking your water?"

"It makes me pee all the time," Dad complained.

"You'll get over that eventually." Sharon always had a smile on her face. "Sign this." She handed him a clipboard.

"What is it?" Dad asked.

"It's the deed to your house," she teased.

"I don't own a house," Dad countered as he signed it.

"Not any more you don't." And off she went, hurrying to her next patient.

Debbie put the probe on Dad's right temple. I could see the machine making pictures of the way his pulse sounded. I had seen it done on television and knew it was supposed to be a sharp up-down beat. Dad's looked like a flattened mountain. Then Debbie put probes on Dad's carotid arteries and pulled two photographs from the ultrasound, one for the right side and one for the left. She compared them to last week's photos. "They look much better," she said, and put them into his file. "Wait for the doctor," she told us.

Dr. Raines showed up a few minutes later. He gave a great bear hug to a patient who was standing in the hall. "You son of a gun! You're looking great!" he bellowed, as he made his way to our station. "Have you noticed any improvement?" he asked Dad.

I was so excited, I burst out first. "Yes. His ankle works better and his toes bend and he is bending his knee when he walks. He can go up the steps to the Institute without stopping, using one leg and then the other."

"Great!" The doctor wrote it all down in big bold strokes.

"He also remembered the name of the flowers I bought. Carnations," I added. "And this morning he used his right hand to butter his toast."

"Look here." Dr. Raines showed Dad and me the two ultrasound pictures that had been taken a week apart. "See how this line goes straight up instead of making an arc? That is an improvement. His blood flow has also dropped from a .58 to a .44 on the right side."

"What does that mean?" Dad asked.

"That is the velocity at which the blood flows. It has reduced. That's good. We need to get rid of those bumps on the left side. It will come."

A nurse entered. "We have him sent to the hospital," she reported quietly to Dr. Raines.

"What happened?" I asked.

"A man had a stroke in the waiting room. We sent him directly to the hospital. He wasn't a patient, yet. He just got here. We hadn't started to medicate him yet."

We were silent for a moment as we each thought about another stroke and the horror of reliving that experience. Forty percent of stroke victims have another stroke within five years. I was thankful that we had begun the medications. Patients on these medications did not have any more strokes. That was a very comforting fact. Not one patient on Dr. Hammesfahr's therapy had had another stroke. It was a remarkable statistic.

"Any questions?" Dr. Raines asked. "No? We are not going to change your medications today. We're done. You can go. See you tomorrow. Drink your water." He raced off to see the next patient. Adorable Debbie waved goodbye.

"Would you carry me out to the car," asked Dad. I burst out laughing. "No, I meant Debbie. Debbie, would you carry me out to the car?"

"He just wants you to put your arms around him, the old lecher!" I cautioned her.

Everyone in the room laughed. The place was full of laughter.

Dad walked out of the clinic without stopping to favor his right foot. I was overjoyed.

A young woman was sitting on the porch. She was thin and had long brown hair. "Oh, you have my shoes!" I exclaimed. She was wearing a pair of blue plastic slides with sunflowers and butterflies on them that appeared and disappeared when the shoes moved. I had on the same silly shoes.

"I love these shoes," she said. "They're happy shoes. They make me laugh." She paused and then burst out crying. "I'm sorry. I am sitting out here crying. I've been crying for the last half an hour," she confessed, holding a handkerchief to her eyes.

"Why are you crying?" I asked, concerned. Everyone in this place was a blithering giggler. I had seen no one cry.

"It's my mother. She had a stroke two and a-half years ago. She'd been in a wheelchair ever since, and she couldn't talk. She had been in the same state all that time. I didn't think she would ever speak again. And now I've had a miracle. My mother just walked up the ramp and into the office." She sobbed and wiped her eyes again. "And this morning, she called me by my name. I never thought I would hear her speak my name again. This is a miracle." She tried to get control of herself. "I just can't stop crying I am so relieved. I am so happy."

Miracle was a word that was tossed around the Institute like confetti. There were dozens of miracles every day. The people in the waiting rooms were bound together like compatriots during a disaster; but these people were partners in a miracle. The staff at the Institute was on the manic side of manic-depressive but never seemed to get to the depressive side. They were so cheerful I sometimes wondered if their emotions were faked. But every time I left, I had a big smile on my face and I felt good. It was a real feeling, not a false one. Getting better was not fake. And it was not a miracle, either. It was the excellent use of medicine. It was the careful observation of patients. It was a doctor who really cared about making people well again.

I started the car. My father began a loud and raunchy version of another song, as we drove down Fort Harrison Avenue. I was glad that the windows were rolled up.

"I'm dancing with tears in my eyes
Cause the girl in my arms isn't you
Dancing with tears in my eyes
When it's you that my heart listens to."

"You are quite a way from dancing with anyone," I commented.

"Yes, but I'm going to. I'm going to." The buoyancy of that place had gotten to him, too. He sang us all the way home.

18
Ironies and Cherries
Thursday, October 12
Day Ten, Medication Day Seven

We were in and out of the Institute fast that morning. But I did remember to bring the magnesium bottle with me. I'd noticed that the directions on the bottle said two tablets a day but the directions the Institute gave me said one tablet. The pharmacist at the drug store substituted the brand, assuring me that it was exactly the same as the one the Institute had prescribed but they apparently could not get. The Institute's instructions said do not substitute drugs. Now I was both substituting and unsure of the dosage. It was amazing to me that something so simple as medication directions could get so confused. I'd done the dose of nitroglycerin cream wrong the first time, using way too much, and then it turned out that I'd given Dad half the dose of magnesium gluconate he should have had. Luckily, at least it was the correct magnesium gluconate.

Directions needed to be reiterated again and again. Each little variation had to be verified. People got the strangest ideas about what they were supposed to do. No wonder the Institute had Educational Sessions every Tuesday and Thursday. The doctors, physical therapist, and educational psychologist took turns talking and answering questions. They spent two-and-a-half-hours discussing major

points and explaining over and over the process, the
medication, and the importance of taking the blood pressure,
drinking the sixty-four ounces of water, and being careful
about what you eat.

"Why is everyone so happy?" Dad asked Sharon as
she hurried by.

She stopped and turned back to look at him. "Is there
something wrong with that?"

"There are two possibilities," Dad said. "You can be
happy or you can be sad. You are always happy."

"Come on, honey," she indicated that we were to
follow her.

"I'm in like Flynn."

"Huh?"

"You called me honey. I'm in luck!" Dad chortled.

Sharon led us to one of the little cubicles with the
three wing chairs. "Sit down here," she said. "I'm going to
take your blood pressure." It was 121/64.

We had a new blood pressure machine to be
calibrated. Sharon told us it was fine. "Now, you must
change the batteries every two weeks, even if the battery
light does not come on."

"Do I have to do this the rest of my life?" Dad asked.

"Yes."

"It sure is a good thing I'm retired. I'd never have
time to do all the things that I have to do for the rest of my
life if I had to work, too."

"Uncross your legs," Sharon said. Dad looked very
sophisticated with his legs crossed. Then I realized that he
had not crossed his legs for years. We had a wonderful
picture of Dad when he was courting mother in the early
1940s. For their fiftieth wedding anniversary we blew it up
huge and put it on the wall at the reception. Dad was sitting
on a rock by the lily pond in the back yard of the Nebraska
farmhouse where mother lived. He had on a two-tone shirt

and racy two-tone shoes. His legs were crossed. He was so handsome. "How come you don't say anything when I cross my arms?" he asked. "You cut off circulation when you cross your legs. We are trying to increase circulation. Don't cross your legs." Sharon had a way of giving orders that made them almost pleasant. I knew she had Dad's best interests at heart. I knew she wanted him to change the way he lived and that is very hard to do. He knew it too.

Dr. Webber arrived and checked the chart. "Your blood sugar is fine. How are you doing?"

"Good. I was a little dizzy last night."

"I gave him three Accupril and didn't give him anything to eat," I said. I think I should give him some food first."

"Absolutely. Woody, eat a snack before you take those pills. You'll do better at night. Any other changes?"

"No."

"Then we'll see you tomorrow."

We were back at the motel before ten.

The far bank of the little stream that ran into the bay had been calling me for the past few days. The four blocks were a long walk for Dad, but it was a cool morning and there was a bench on the other end where he could sit and rest. "Let's take a walk," I suggested. "Do you think you can make it across the river?'

"I can't swim it," he joked.

"How about taking the sidewalk?"

"Let's try it." We began walking slowly. "My leg hurts a little this morning."

"Is it brain pain or is it muscle pain?"

"It's not like anything I've felt before. My leg tingles like there are little prickly points up and down it."

"Maybe that is healing. Before you couldn't feel much, now you can feel things." It didn't seem like an unreasonable idea to me.

My youngest son, Bradley, had called from Los Angeles the night before. He had been working on a pilot for a new TV show. He went around LA asking people who they would like to change places with for a week. Whose lifestyle would they like to experience? "What do you think you would answer to that?" I asked Dad.

"I don't know," he said thoughtfully. "I like my life. I wouldn't change."

"A child answered that he would like to change places with his teacher but most of the older people said that they would rather keep their lives as they were. Think about it, Dad. You've had a stroke. Wouldn't you like to exchange lives with someone who hasn't had a stroke? Bradley said he would like to exchange with Hugh Hefner."

"He's just young. His hormones are raging." Dad thought about it for a minute. "I've had a really good life. I wouldn't exchange it. Besides, the other person would have to be in my body. I wouldn't want that." He was thoughtful for a while as we walked slowly back across the bridge.

A horn beeped at us. It was Daniel, the young man from England. He was driving a blue convertible with the top down. He waved with his arm high above his head as he drove past.

Our afternoon appointment was with the educational psychologist, Timothy. "I'm going to talk to you for about an hour this afternoon," he said, as he walked us down the narrow hall.

"An hour?" said Dad. "I better go to the bathroom first." He turned off at the bathroom.

"Sixty-four ounces of water a day," I said. "It goes though a person fast. Did you bring your writing for me?" Timothy had approached me to look at his writing on out last visit. As I had taught writing for many years and felt confident in my abilities to advise young writers, I'd agreed.

"No, I forgot."

"Ah. Fear." He would have remembered if he had not been afraid that I would judge harshly.

Once, in high school, I showed my writing to a trusted and much-admired teacher. The first thing she said was, "You've made some spelling mistakes."

"I'll correct them," I muttered, as I took the paper and left.

I never read that paper again, although I kept it in my folder for the whole year. I never corrected the spelling mistakes, but I learned a valuable teaching lesson. Praise first. Criticize later. Discuss the ideas, the beauty of the language, and the sensitivity of the writing. As an afterthought, you might mention the spelling. Now, any computer can do that mechanical job. Only creative humans can write poems or tell stories.

It is fear that keeps people from trying new things like Dr. Hammesfahr's therapy. They deny that they could improve before they know anything about the therapy for fear that it won't work. They don't want to raise their hopes because they are afraid of the disappointment if they fail to improve.

"You need courage, Timothy." I said. "Either you are afraid that the subject matter is too emotional or you are afraid that you are not a good writer."

"I'm not a good writer. That's for sure."

"There you go."

"I'll bring it next time I see you. I promise."

"I'll expect it."

We settled into comfortable chairs as dad came back into the room.

"I just want you to tell me about yourself," Timothy began. "Any signs of improvement?"

"My arm hurts less," said Dad.

"It hurts less?" Timothy repeated, in his best Carl Rogers counseling style. My father had taught me years ago the technique of echoing the last sentence a person said. It worked every time to get the other person talking.

"And less in my leg when my daughter doesn't walk me all over creation," Dad said.

"Are you going to the meeting this afternoon?"

"Yes."

"Where is it?"

"In that place where the water is. I know where, just a minute. That place by the water, the Yacht Club."

"Are you remembering more?"

"Yes, I think my brain is functioning better. It's nice to have it back. Since the doctor's been filling me with drugs I'm remembering things I'd forgotten for years. I'm almost ready to start living again."

"What did you do?"

"I did some very interesting research in your field," Dad said. "I gave aptitude tests, verbal, numerical, abstract, spatial, and mechanical, to every student who entered the university. In the course of my counseling work I discovered that there was a relationship between the kinds of problems the kids were coming into my office with, and the kind of test scores they had. For instance, I got so good at reading the test results that I could predict, before I ever talked to a student, the general emotional problem that student would present to me. A student with a low verbal score and higher other scores would talk about guilt. A student with a low abstract score would talk to me about problems of self-worth. It seemed crazy, but it worked. I never got to prove the theory, but it was fascinating." Dad shifted in his chair.

"I had a good friend on campus who was a physician, and the university was just starting to use computers. We began to run a correlation between the test results and the kind of complaints that students brought to the health clinic. For instance, students with low verbal scores complained of respiratory problems, while students with low abstract scores came in with stomach ailments. I wish I had finished that research."

"There are two good research problems for you, Timothy," I said. "My father is brilliant."

"I guess so. You are full of interesting hypotheses, Woody."

"Dad also builds houses. And he is an extraordinary Thespian. He acts and directs, and he ran the Community Theater. He did everything from balancing the books to fixing the roof."

"Oh Robin, cut it out. I don't deserve it," Dad laughed.

"And he can sing. Want to hear him?"

We sang, "Life is just a bowl of cherries," again and this time he knew the words and sang them loudly. He put special emphasis on "You can't take your dough when you go, go, go." I knew he was thinking of the $590 he had paid to let Timothy listen to him sing.

"He's helped my children too, especially my two boys."

"How did you do that?"

"Her son got a big part in a TV series. He was Mary Tyler Moore's son in 'Annie McGuire.' My wife and I took him to California so he could live there and make the episodes. Robin was still teaching," Dad said.

"That's not all. Dad did a lot of counseling while he was out there. I'm divorced. Both my boys had problems with the break-up."

"I made an effort," he said. "Her older boy came and lived with me while he went to graduate school to get a master's degree in computer programming.

"Dad helped my older son, who was struggling and didn't have a job, get back on track, too."

"You must have changed a lot of people's lives."

"Oh no. I didn't change any lives. I gave them the opportunity to change their own lives. They had to choose to do that."

"You are a humble man."

"I never thought of myself that way. I was given a gift, a good brain. I just used it."

"You and your daughter are very close."

"I have two daughters. I am close to both of them." Timothy leaned forward in his seat.

"I can see by the way he is sitting that he's earned his money," Dad said. "Time to go, Robin."

"I'll remember to bring my writing when I see you again," Timothy said, as he led us out of the office. "This has been a fascinating hour."

We climbed back into the little green car.

"You were stupendous, Dad!"

"What do you think he'll write about me?"

"That you are witty and intelligent, and a great thinker, and a wise man."

"Pshaw! If I'm that great why aren't I well."

"A wise man with a stroke," I added, as we head off towards the Thursday Educational Session.

Donna began the session with a positive statement. "So many people are concentrating on what's wrong with them I thought today we would celebrate the things that we have. Here are Harry and Lorraine. Say a few words."

"My wife had a stroke last January twenty-fifth. She was in the hospital twenty-one days and in rehab for two months. The doctors told us that was all the return she was going to get. I saw a brochure for the Institute at my tax man's office. We were drowning, so I was clutching at straws and I followed up on the brochure. Now she can walk with a cane and speak much better."

"How did you find out about this treatment?" Donna asked another couple.

"Sheryl and I were at a Heart Association Meeting. The man in the next chair told me about it. He gave me the phone number."

A striking Swedish woman said she'd found the ad in an airline magazine. "There must have been a lot of people who tore that ad out," she said. "I asked my neurologist about it. He didn't know anything about the therapy, but he said, 'You go. Come back and tell me about it.' I can't wait to go home to tell him."

"Most doctors are deaf, dumb, and blind when it comes to new things," a caregiver commented. "You were lucky your neurologist said to go."

"My wife had a stroke ten years ago," said a man who introduced himself as James. "The doctors said she had everything back that she was ever going to get back. Baloney! We're here for our three-month check-up. Now she walks a mile at a time. When we walk around the shopping mall in winter, I carry a pack of Dr. Hammesfahr's cards. Whenever we see other stroke victims we stop and talk and give them cards. I'm not shy about stopping perfect strangers to hand out the cards."

They were sitting with another couple. "We're among those who got the card from these two strangers in the mall," the wife said. "And we just happen to be here at the Institute at the same time."

"We heard about Dr. Hammesfahr on a radio talk show," another man said. "Dawn couldn't walk at all. She had seizures. Now she can talk better and she can walk six or seven hundred feet all by herself, and she no longer has seizures."

A heavy-set man with curly hair said, "I haven't had much of a change because I just started medications last week. But I have had one major improvement. Since the stroke, I had not been able to sleep lying down in a bed. I had to sleep sitting up in a chair because I got a severe case of vertigo whenever I lay down. Last night, I slept lying down in a bed for the first time in five years."

The audience applauded. "Vertigo is vertigone," quipped Kate, a woman obviously fond of words.

Jenny's husband spoke next. "There was no dramatic change, just gradual improvement. She likes to go to the beauty shop to get her hair fixed. A year ago I had to help her. Now she goes by herself. When we began the treatment, I had to take her to the washroom. That was really awkward. Now, she can do it on her own. I know she will speak again."

"This is a very interesting case," Dr. Hammesfahr commented, "because two years ago I thought that Jenny might be one of our few failures. She could not speak. She did not have any immediate recovery. Now, two years later, we find that the medications have been working all along, just slowly."

A fellow named Dave said, "I saw the palm of my hand for the first time in eight years, and I am now able to move my fingers." He stretched his fingers out to demonstrate.

"I can turn over in bed," a tall thin woman said. "Before, the afflicted side was so heavy I couldn't move it."

"I see change overnight. New improvements often happen in the morning," another patient added.

"The pain in my face is gone," said a flirtatious white-haired man. "Blood brings back use to parts of me that I thought I would never use again." He winked, salaciously. "I got my golf swing back, too." Dad offered his cane and the jovial gentleman swung it like a golf club from his right shoulder all the way around to complete a back swing, almost hitting a woman nearby in his enthusiasm.

"My husband had a stroke in 1997," said a dark-haired woman named Helen. "He is much improved mentally now. He is happy-go-lucky. Before he was depressed. The physical changes have been more subtle, but steady."

The man who'd had to buy shoes in two different sizes spoke next. "I'm coming back after six months. I've had gradual improvement. My hand can go flat again. Now I can clap and open a door."

"I'm not good at putting on my socks, but I'm getting real good at shooting them across the room while trying," said George, a teacher from California.

"He's not so good at picking them up," said his wife. "It' more like, 'Linda, come get my socks.'"

"I prayed that God would enlighten someone to help my husband," the Swedish woman said, as Dr. Hammesfahr came to the front of the room. "He enlightened you, and I found you." Everyone applauded in agreement. "Thank you Almighty Creator," the woman said.

"Thank you. Thank you very much," Dr. Hammesfahr said. "I'm kind of embarrassed about all this. We do start every day with a prayer meeting. God chose a strange place for all this to be discovered. While this treatment may be the result of enlightenment, it was also the result of a lot of hard work."

It did not look as though he convinced many people in the room.

"I want everyone to know that even though I am not able to see every patient every day any more, I still see all the files. My staff is getting really good results. We think that more doctors working on each case improves the care for the patient. When we advertised three positions on our staff, we had more than a thousand applications. The three we chose are superb physicians. One of them has been president of the Florida State Osteopathic Medical Society twice. We all work very closely together.

"Our patients get better, but it does take time. We have millions of nerves in our bodies, not just one. It takes time for a group of these to heal. First, we begin to see the side effects of small improvements in the blood flow to the brain. For instance, a person might have a lyric response first, and then sounds, before he says a single word. But if you see a small response that means the brain is beginning to heal in that area. That is where you should look for further healing. If you stop having any improvement for more than three months, come back here. Every year people get better and better. It's not always like a sudden awakening, it's gradual. The key is to stick with it. If you stop drinking water, you will have trouble."

Dr. Hammesfahr was standing beside an easel with a big drawing tablet on it. He was wearing scuffed loafers and his feet were curled one over the other like a little boy's. His slacks and jacket were casual and rumpled. His pale blue shirt matched his eyes. He was full of energy and passion. He spoke without notes, from the heart. He answered every question with candor and perception.

"All of you who have a stroke are here because your caregivers got you here and through the initial phase. Give them a break. Send them out twice a week for an afternoon. And caretakers, be sure to give yourselves time alone. You need to last for the long haul.

"Stroke patients who still have a living spouse who will care for them are the lucky ones. Many others move into retirement homes. Their children, if they have had them, have full time jobs. Of course they stop in to see them, but even the ones who live in the same town can not be there for the constant needs of a stroke patient.

"Families try to overcome this, but they are hindered by the depression of the stroke patient. When the families think that they are doing the best thing for the patient, the patient often misinterprets this as "running their lives" or "losing control." Depression enhances the negative aspects of these feelings. This is an emotional response and while they often they realize intellectually that their families are trying to do the best thing, emotionally they are still resentful.

"Does everyone have to come for three weeks?"

"When we first started this treatment we administered it over the course of a year. Now we do it in three weeks and it works better because it works faster. "One of our first patients had had a stroke thirty-seven years before, a childhood stroke. He got the use of his hand back within six to eight months. We must teach you a new life style. You must follow the rules and watch carefully. More things can happen three months or six months down the road. Medication doses can change.

"All of you from all around the country are ambassadors for this therapy. We want to establish support groups in different parts of the country, and identify doctors in different areas who will help with the therapy. If you are interested in being in a support group, please give your name to Donna." Dr. Hammesfahr paused and looked around the room.

Karen, a small young woman who had been in a car accident, raised her hand. She was in a wheelchair, had lost the use of one hand, and could not walk. Her speech was slurred and difficult to understand. She looked very angry. "When will I get rid of the pain?" she demanded.

"Most patients get rid of thalamic pain in six to nine months," Dr. Hammesfahr said. "With car injuries, neck nerves that control the brain are damaged. That affects concentration, balance, headaches and strokes. But it does not show up on an MRI.

"Pain usually lessens in five or six months. As a rule of thumb, in anything that begins to work, you can expect twenty percent improvement the first year. Nerves repair themselves over time. A damaged nerve that has short-circuited causes pain. The pain comes with anything that is not totally dead. If a nerve is alive, its chance of getting better is excellent. It just takes time. It's a different kind of pain. You'll be able to tell the difference."

"Can I do aerobic exercises?" Karen asked. "I want to keep my body strong." She looked defiantly at her parents sitting next to her. "Overheating the body is bad. If you get too much medicine or if you get too hot, blood rushes to your feet and away from your brain. The amount of medication you can tolerate can fluctuate with the full moon, the seasons, changes in temperature, or changes in altitude."

It occurred to me that maybe the reason Dad had had a slow start was that cold morning we had.

Dr. Hammesfahr continued, "Salt consumption, hormones, arthritis in the neck, water, artificial sweeteners, coffee, and alcohol affect it. That's why it is important to keep your blood pressure in the target range. It means that you are keeping your blood vessels the right size. Everything in moderation. Not too large and not to too small. If your blood pressure is too high or too low you don't improve. Watch your blood pressure. Stay in your target range.

"When you exercise, your medications get out of whack and you may fall or get hurt. The physical therapist who urges you to try harder is doing you a disservice. The rule is, don't force it. Be observant. Notice what time of day you do better. Improvement is faster if you are not erratic.

"Look for weather-related changes. Reduce the medication in the summer and increase it in the winter. Ninety percent of you will be making your own adjustments inside of a year. That just happens."

"What about Mexican pharmacies?"

"It's the same medication, only its twenty cents on the dollar. You can order it on the Internet and they will mail it to you. Every other country in the world has cheaper medicine than the United States."

"Why won't Medicare pay for this?"

"That is beyond me. They did for five years. There is one doctor here in Florida, who sets the rules for Medicare. He has denied the claims. Write to your Senators and

Representatives. I am working as hard as I can to get that changed, because I do not want this to be a treatment for the rich only."

Question after question came pouring in from the audience. The room was full of energy, which seemed odd since half the people in it had some form of what they had thought was a permanent disability. In another place, a room like that might have reminded me of Dad's retirement home, the Fort Armstrong Hotel, where the lobby was sometimes full of people, all dozing. There were cheerful people working at the home, but many of the residents seemed totally without hope, waiting to die. Here, people were excited. They were filled with the possibility that they could get better. There was something they could do, rather than prepare to die.

"We're going to have a newsletter and a web site for the Institute. It will be HNI-Online.com" Dr. Hammesfahr said. "We've made a lot of changes in the last year. Things change pretty often here."

It was five o'clock. The session had whizzed by. Dr. Hammesfahr had said that Dad's pain would be gone in nine months. Nine months seemed like a long time, but I was sure that nine months later, that time would have whizzed by, too.

19

The Thirteenth

Friday, October 13

Day Eleven, Medication Day Eight

Dr. Raines rushed through the waiting room just as we were arriving at the clinic for our appointment to get a magnesium shot and talk to a doctor. "How are you?" he asked Dad. "Any recovery?"

"None," answered dad. "I haven't seen any."

"That's ridiculous," I said. "What do you mean, none? What about all that stuff you told me yesterday?"

Dad looked confused.

"He can do lots of things better. His leg is better, and he can climb stairs more easily, and he thinks a lot better. He did a brilliant tour de force at the educational psychologist's office yesterday."

"Often the patient doesn't see the changes that are occurring," Dr. Raines said. "That is why it's important for the caregiver to make notes on what has changed. A lot of people are not observant. I talked to a man who was leaving a few days ago and he said, 'I really can't do anything better, but now I have hope that I will.' However, he was already much better. He could move his hand and bend his ankle. There are some people who do not get better, but very, very few."

I made a note to ask Dr. Hammesfahr about the very, very, few.

"The neurologists in Florida think that this therapy couldn't possibly work." Dr. Raines continued. "But no one has a corner on knowledge. Many things were discovered by serendipity – penicillin, Viagra, the antibiotics that cure ulcers. They were all serendipitous occurrences. Dr. Hammesfahr is an idea man. He just said, 'I wonder if...?' and it worked."

"Why did you come to work at the Institute?" I asked.

"I had been a doctor for thirty-five years and was planning to retire. Dr. Hammesfahr and I had known each other for the past ten years. When he began this therapy, I thought it wouldn't be successful, but since I was going to retire I sent him a bunch of stroke patients and they all got better. He was wildly successful. Then he said, 'Why don't you come to work for me?' and I did."

"This is some retirement," Dad said. "You are always running through here."

"That's my normal pace. I've always been a fast mover," he said, as Sharon zoomed by. "The workers here are so upbeat, it's amazing. Where did you ever see such happiness?"

When Sharon returned she moved us into the back room and took Dad's blood pressure. It was 162/72.

The couple next to us was talking about their doctor in Pembroke Pines. "We called him and asked him what to do and he said. 'I really don't know. Why don't you call Dr. Hammesfahr? Let me know what he says.' That was it. I thought if I'm going to call him, I don't need you. We dropped him and now we drive 250 miles every two weeks to see Dr. Hammesfahr. It's worth it."

It was another tale of uncooperative doctors. "This art, or science, of medicine sure has a lot of doctors who think that their way is the only way of doing things," I commented to Dad. Dr. Webber came over and began looking at Dad's charts.

"That is true of all professions. You can get along very well if you don't have any ideas," Dad said, directly to him.

"Right!" Dr. Webber guffawed. It was the first time I had seen him truly affected by anything we had said. He was so soft spoken and shy that his secret nickname among the patients was Elmer Fudd. He must have tried to change the world and been outspoken at one time, because he surely understood the concept.

"It's certainly true of teachers," I said. "I tried to convince teachers that using the arts to teach in their areas of expertise would make it easier for students to learn. I felt as though I was fighting them every inch of the way."

"All teachers with ideas have to fight for them," Dr. Webber said.

"That is probably why I retired. I just got tired of trying to change people who had no desire to change. Now I'm working on changing myself. That's enough of a challenge."

Dr. Webber asked Dad if he had noticed any changes.

"My leg hurts. It's a prickly sensation," dad complained.

"Good," the doctor said. "Sensation is returning to the leg." He wrote it down.

"First time I heard pain was good," Dad muttered, crossing his legs.

"See what he is doing? When was the last time you crossed your legs, Dad?" I turned to Dr. Webber. "Last week he couldn't cross his legs."

"It cuts off your circulation if you cross your legs, Dr. Robinson." Stay on the same medication over the weekend. We'll see you on Monday."

Sharon came to give Dad his injection of magnesium gluconate. "Uncross your legs, Woody."

Dad did so and immediately re-crossed them in the opposite direction. Sharon put her hands on her hips and crinkled her nose as he laughed at his own joke and uncrossed his legs again.

"Watch me do this," she told me. "You will have to do it when you get home."

"Oh, no I won't. I live in Chicago and he lives in Rock Island. He will have to have his doctor do it." I watched her anyway.

"Jab them in the fatty tissue." She had two needles full of clear liquid that she injected into Dad's rump. "Nice fat!" she remarked.

About ten seconds later, Dad said. "Ouch!"

"You faker," she teased.

"I don't even know if I have a doctor," Dad worried. I've never seen him. I hope he takes me as a patient when I get home."

"He will. He said he would. Dr. Flowers comes twice a week to Dad's retirement home," I said.

"That should be okay. He can do it then." Sharon hurried off.

Dr. Uzo sped by in her Dr. Scholl's sandals and her red toenail polish. "Are you doing well today, Woody?" she asked, as we rose to leave.

"As well as can be expected," Dad said.

20
Flying with Possibilities
Saturday, October 14
Day Twelve, Medication Day Nine

The morning dawned with a brilliant blue sky. Dad had rearranged the magnetic letters on the side of the refrigerator to say U LOVE I a few days before, and he pointed it out to me.

"That's the truth, Robin. You have done a wonderful thing for me by bringing me here." He was eating his breakfast and grinning.

"That's a good reason to drive down to Clearwater Beach for lunch. It will give me a break from fixing meals. There's probably a place right on the beach where we can wiggle our toes in the sand and eat a fish sandwich. We won't sit in the room all day."

We took Fort Harrison Drive to the turnoff to the beach. It was very hot when we got out of the car and walked a block to the café. Yellow umbrellas stood in two lines up and down the beach, with wooden chairs set out under them. It looked like a postcard.

But the café was a stand-up counter for take-out. That would be impossible for Dad to manage. "We can't eat here. Let's just sit awhile," I suggested.

Dad had walked two blocks in the bright sun. That was probably not the best move on my part. He had been warned to keep from overexerting or getting too hot, as that would affect his blood pressure. Too much physical exercise was bad for him. I certainly didn't want him to loose his balance and fall. The doctors and nurses had cautioned us against trying to do too much once Dad felt better.

"You know," he said, "I sleep so much at home because I don't have anything to do. Monday I read the mail and pay the bills. Then I sleep in the afternoon for a couple of hours. In the evening, I play bridge. Tuesday is an empty day and I sleep in the morning and in the afternoon. Wednesday evening I play bridge again. Thursday, I play bridge all day. Saturday, I have nothing to do and there is no good TV. I usually go to your sister's house on Sunday afternoon, but I hate to impose on them, taking their Sundays every week."

"Now that you are feeling better, why don't you do some volunteering? You're still a great psychologist. You could counsel stroke patients and their caregivers."

"How would I go about doing that?"

"There must be an organization in Rock Island. Ask the nurse at the Fort Armstrong. She might know of one. Ask your new doctor."

He nodded.

"You could sing," I suggested.

"Where?"

Mother always joined a church first thing, every time we moved. We moved every year, so there were a lot of new churches. She said that church members have to be friendly and nice to you because they're good Christians. She used to joke, "It's the only hour in the week that no one asks me to do anything."

I understood the feeling. As a teacher, most of my day was spent doing things for other people. Having an hour simply to think and contemplate was a prized gift. But mother had other reasons for going to church on Sunday morning. As I grew older, I realized that she enjoyed the rituals of the service. There was comfort for her in the repetitive pattern, in singing the hymns to which she knew all the words.

Dad often sang in the choirs and sometimes Mother joined him. She had a weak scrawny voice with uncertain pitch, but she sang with gusto. When there was a choirmaster with pretensions, she was occasionally asked not to sing during certain sensitive parts.

"You could join a church choir. They always need a strong bass."

"I can't read the words fast enough to sing them," Dad said.

"Join a Lutheran Church and you will already know all the words. You've sung in enough Lutheran choirs to know all the hymns by heart."

"I would like to sing," he confessed.

"You could always sing boo-be-boo-be-boo, like Ella Fitzgerald. Or sing, I forgot the line, but I think it's gonna rhyme."

"I might look into it."

We left the bench when the sun got too hot and drove down the beach road. We crossed an incredible bridge between Clearwater Beach and Sand Island in the Gulf of Mexico. It had been built to allow tall boats to pass underneath and it was huge. We started up the incline, pointing the nose of our little green Sunfire into the blue sky. We might get to the top of that bridge and keep on going into the sky. Maybe we could even fly. We could be our own Sunfire. We were full of ourselves and our possibilities for the future. Coming down was a slippery-slide thrill. We started the descent without a thought of turning back.

The bridge delivered us into the arms of the Columbia Restaurant. We made our way through the bar to a row of tables with umbrellas on a sunny deck overlooking a sailboat race. It was a perfect day. Dad was going to be able to do many new things. Life was very good. So was lunch.

When I got home I sent an e-mail to everyone.

Dear Friends and Relatives,

We are on Day Twelve of our odyssey. Dad has been on his medications for nine days. He has already seen improvement in his thinking skills. I can see that he no longer struggles for words or ideas. I no longer hear, "Darn it, I can't remember that. I give up." He is coherent and witty. That would be enough as far as I am concerned. It is such a miracle that he can think again.

But there's more good news. The screeching pain that he felt each time he took a step is gone. He is getting feeling back in his right leg. He can bend his knee when he walks, and his ankle and toe bend, as well. These are excellent signs, as once repair works starts on the portion of his brain that controls his leg and foot they will continue to get better.

Miracles abound in this place like confetti. Patients who have been told that they will never get any better are getting better. Dad has lived with that downer for eight years. To see his improvement right before my eyes is amazing. Everyone gets better. Some people do so in the first week, others in second week. Almost everyone shows improvement by the third week. You know, I didn't realize how depressing doctors' offices were until I spent time in Dr. Hammesfahr's waiting room and saw the joy in all of the people sitting there.

I have great stories from everyone I meet here.

There is hope! Tell everyone!

Celebrate with us tonight, with a toast to all creative people who struggle against a disbelieving world. I am in the middle of what seems like a miracle. But it is not. It is the dedicated practice of medicine from an intelligent, gifted man.

Love, Robin

21
Follow the Golden Road
Sunday, October 15
Day Thirteen, Medication Day Ten

In the past few years I have developed a passion for beauty. It is odd because I always thought intelligence, or enthusiasm, or persistence were the important things in my life. Aside from the occasional sunset while on vacation, beauty never caught my eye. Now, I watch skies and water and birds. On that Sunday morning I spent ten minutes looking at the shadows of a bush blowing in the breeze. I saw my feathered friend, an American oyster catcher, at the edge of the canal. He was a black and white bird with yellow legs and a big bright red beak. I put a plastic chair behind the motel and waited for him daily, checking tides in the local paper. I watched him work the oyster beds that lined the edges of the canal. Early that morning, I also saw a group of rare white pelicans with black wing tips, flying overhead. The light glistening on the water made me want to hold my breath and preserve the moment. It was a kind of worship.

On our walk from the Aloha Motel out to the fishing pier on Clearwater Bay that day, I was surprised to see people wading hundreds of yards off shore. They were only knee-deep in water. I guess I should have realized that the water was so shallow, as I had seen birds feeding far out in the bay, but it did not register until I saw the humans. Some were throwing huge round nets like the "National Geographic" pictures of Southeast Asians fishing in rice paddies. Others carried buckets. I had no idea what they were doing.

Dad had walked out to the farthest pier with me, and he sat in the lawn chair gazing at the horizon.

"The medicine is having an effect," he said. "I'm feeling a heck of a lot different. My leg doesn't hurt as much as it did. I can walk without screeching pain with every step. My foot seems to move better, and my ankle and toes bend when I step."

"Big changes."

"It's a little scary," he said as we walked back to the motel. "I'm not sure I trust it. I'm not sure that if I step down on my foot the whole leg won't go out from underneath me. I'm afraid my knee is going to give out."

"Maybe the muscles are weak there," I suggested. "If the muscles are weak, you could feel as though you might fall over whenever you took a step."

"Could be," he agreed.

Later that morning we drove down to Bradenton to keep our lunch date with Brooks and Dorothy. Their daughter, Heather, the victim of an accident sixteen years before, had been rushed to the emergency room a few days earlier with a seizure or maybe the flu. They were worried about it happening again. I thought about the terror that my mother's seizures had brought to Dad and Lia. I wanted to see Brooks and Dorothy of course, but I really wanted to see them in order to talk face to face about Dr. Hammesfahr.

To get to their house we crossed a new five-mile bridge on highway US 275. A barge had run into the old bridge and damaged it. The new one was high enough to allow large ships to pass beneath it. Brooks had told me it was beautiful, but that did not prepare me for the huge upsweep of the road that sent us skyward. At the center of the bridge golden suspension wires swooped up to spires and then down again on the other side. They called it the Sunshine Bridge.

Dorothy had misgivings about partially curing Heather. I empathized with her and Brooks. They had total responsibility for another human being and that carried with it a terrible weight.

I told Dad what they'd said and he harrumphed.

"Well, what do you mean by that?" I said.

"They don't have a right to decide for their daughter. They have to do what they think will help her the most."

"But they have to take care of her. What if she is miserable or angry and demanding?"

"What if she isn't? What if she is grateful and full of love and brings them joy?"

"I suppose that is a chance they'd have to take," I mused.

"That's the chance all parents take. They do the best that they can for their children. Then they react to whatever situations arise. If Heather is depressed, she will deal with depression, and her parents can help. If she is angry, she will have to work through the anger. Lots of people do. I call that living."

"Still, it is a hard decision for them to make." I didn't know if they even wanted to talk about it. They had not pulled up the web site on the Internet.

But there was the bridge, the second golden road on this trip. I could not help but think it was a sign that I was on the right path and that I should convince them to investigate this possibility of treatment for Heather.

Brooks and Dorothy were in great spirits when we arrived. They had set the table on the patio near the pool and it looked elegant and delightful. Brooks no longer had circles under his eyes. Dorothy had a healthy glow.

"How's retirement?" I asked.

"We are on a permanent vacation," Brooks declared.

We got a tour of their lovely ranch house. Heather was in the kitchen. Dorothy introduced her to Dad. Heather eyed me up and down and shifted her focus to him.

He smiled. "Hi Heather," he said.

Heather's face lit up as she stared at my father, flirting.

"She likes you," Dorothy told Dad. "She likes men a lot."

As we moved outside to the seating area next to the pool, Dad said privately, "She scared me a little. I thought she was going to jump into my lap."

"She did look eager, but she can't move, dad," I whispered. "You're safe,"

Dorothy and Brooks lit cigarettes. "Do you mind if we smoke? We don't smoke in the house, so we spend most of our time outside."

"No, I don't mind. Dad smoked for sixty years before his stroke."

"I know we shouldn't, but we just can't stop."

"Dr. Hammesfahr wouldn't approve."

"We have been talking to people about this Institute," Dorothy said. "No one seems to know anything about it. The internal medicine guy who treated Heather when she was in the hospital this week gave us his card and said that if we went to the Institute, he would be happy to work with us afterwards. He was very open to new ideas."

"That's worth something." I said. "Not every doctor is."

"We have been hunting for a GP since we got down here in July, but we haven't found one yet. The problem with the doctor we saw this week is he's foreign and difficult to understand. And I wanted a woman physician for Heather and me."

"The Institute has a list of doctors who are cooperating already," I said. "Maybe you can find one of those."

"The problem is that Medicare doesn't cover it," Brooks said.

"It is expensive. It cost us $6,000 up front. But at least you live down here and can make day trips for the treatment. We are also spending $3,000 more on plane tickets, car rental, and motel, not to mention eating. I sure wish Dad's insurance would pay for it."

"Heather's accident caused overall damage to the whole brain," Dorothy said. "She was without oxygen for twenty minutes or so. She has brain stem injury. I don't know if Dr. Hammesfahr can be of help in a situation like that."

"I don't know, either."

"We did a labor intensive program with Heather in Philadelphia for more than seven years that employed patterning. That's when we used the volunteers. Over the years we've had hundreds of volunteers. We just saw one of them. He was a man who used to come down from the north shore to help. He recently had a stroke. I should tell him about this place."

Dorothy went into a long explanation of how the patterning worked. It involved repeating actions over and over again in the hope that a different section of Heather's brain would take over for the damaged sections and she would be able to move again. Dorothy rose from her chair. "Would you like wine with lunch?"

"I would, but I have to drive back, so I better not have any. Dad isn't allowed to drink any kind of alcohol. It constricts the blood vessels."

"Decaffeinated iced tea?"

"Fine."

"I'll have water," Dad said. He was working on his sixty-four ounces a day. Tea did not count as water, and decaffeinated tea and coffee were on the 'No' list, anyway.

Lunch was lovely. Heather's nurse took her on a long walk and we did not see her again before we had to leave so we'd have time to get home before dark.

"We're going to try to come up to Clearwater to check out the Institute," Brooks said. "I would like to get there before you guys leave."

"Education Sessions are Tuesday and Thursday afternoons from two-thirty to four-thirty." I said. "That's when I think you should come. You can ask all the questions you want at these sessions. The doctors, the psychologist, and the physical therapist are all there."

"When are you leaving?" Dorothy asked.

"On the 24th."

"Have a good drive back," Brooks said. They stood side-by-side in the driveway and waved as we pulled out, looking like a contemporary version of "American Gothic."

I was tired on the way home and had to open the window to keep the fresh air on my face. We were back at the motel by six. I made Dad a sandwich and we both watched TV, exhausted.

I thought about our day and about miracles and why people rejected them. Perhaps they didn't want to change because change was difficult, even a change for the better required complex adjustments in behavior and lifestyle. Maybe, like my sister, they were too worn out from a previous traumatic experience or they were afraid things would get worse instead of better, like Brooks and Dorothy. As Dad kept saying, "It's not easy, this getting well again."

But Brooks and Dorothy had said they would visit the Institute, so I hoped that their first reaction would not be their last.

22
Hubris/Pride
Monday, October 16
Day Fourteen, Medication Day Eleven

I woke up at six-thirty with an awful thought. I had forgotten to give Dad his three Accupril and the Nitro cream last night. I'd sent him to bed without his medication. The sole reason I was down here was to look after Dad. Making sure that he took his medications was my main job, and I had failed. What was the matter with me? How could I have been so negligent? The evening dose was his heaviest. To skip that dose was to defeat the purpose of being here. I did a little self-flagellation while I brushed my teeth.

We had gotten too tired the day before. I'd fallen asleep in front of TV before Dad did. Then when I awoke I found him sleeping in his chair and sent him to bed before I staggered to my bedroom. I totally forgot that he had to have medicine and some food. So did he. We were not going to get that tired again. I would have to see to it that our days were less full.

We had made the same mistake that many patients did when they started getting better – they overexerted with physical activities that were far beyond their capabilities. They tried to dance or to take long walks and fell down and injured themselves. Dad's brain had improved and we tried to use it too much. It was the intellectual version of tap dancing or aerobics.

As for myself, I had no excuse. I should not have grown tired with a day's activities. I should have remembered Dad's medicine. Guilt was what I deserved for getting cocky and thinking subconsciously that everything was fine.

I asked Dad the morning questions, the day, year, month, his location, and who was president of the United States. I took his blood pressure, 119/64. The diastolic was low.

I didn't want show my face at the doctor's office that morning but we had a nine-fifty appointment. The parking lot was deserted and so was the waiting room. Five or six patients were there ahead of us, but they all had been seen already. We were taken right into the room with the big wing chairs. Sharon took Dad's blood pressure. It was 126/68, close to perfect.

"Dr. Webber," I asked with feigned casualness, "what does he do if he misses pills? Does he take extra ones when we discover the error?"

The doctor responded in his usual gentle manner. "No, don't worry if his blood pressure is still in the acceptable range. You should do something if it is out of the range for a few days, or if there are symptoms such as dizziness or disorientation. But one missed dose doesn't make a big difference. The medicine builds up in his system."

"I forgot to give him his pills last night," I confessed. "I feel so guilty for missing those pills. It was simply hubris. Too much pride. We did too much and we got too tired. I thought we were on the way to recovery and I got careless with our energy. My arrogance was punished. I am the caretaker. I am not allowed to make mistakes."

"You're human," Dr. Webber said.

"Don't be too hard on yourself," Dad added.

I knew that they didn't blame me, but I still felt terrible. When we got back to the motel I planned to recheck all of his dosages and put them into a little plastic pillbox that we had purchased the week before. It was divided into days and then morning, noon, evening, and bedtime. Maybe if I made the process of figuring out what to take easier, we could concentrate on taking it on time.

We saw Nancy and Dirk, the couple from Colorado, on our way out of the office. Dirk was smiling and talking to his wife.

"You look pretty chipper," I said.

"He can say short sentences! He had this stroke ten years ago and he hasn't been much of a conversationalist since then. Now he is my conversational companion again." She poked him playfully.

"How long has he been on medication?" I asked. I had spoken to Nancy five days before, when she and Dirk first arrived at the Institute. He had been disinterested and disconnected from the conversation.

"He's not even on Accupril yet, because his blood pressure is too low. This is just from nitroglycerin cream and magnesium."

"And that made him speak? Remarkable! Aren't you glad that stranger handed you that phone number at the Bingo game?"

"I am amazed at how that happened to us. I thank the Lord every day for sending us the money to come here."

I imagined myself walking through the mall and stopping stroke victims to hand out Dr. Hammesfahr's cards. Not trying to convince them, just saying, "Do you want this card? This man can heal you."

I watched my father's favorite programs on TV each night during the weeks we spent together. "Diagnosis Murder," "Walker, Texas Ranger," "Touched by an Angel," "Murder She Wrote," and "Early Edition" were his favorites. The one that intrigued me the most was about angels. They appeared in each program with a miracle to hand out. In one show, the angels tried to get people to accept a miracle. Some people just said no, others wanted to hand the miracle off to someone else, but no one took the miracle for himself.

I knew there would be stroke victims like that. There would be people who would see Dad's recovery and still not take the risk necessary to come to Clearwater and recover from their own strokes. It took courage to change.

Later that evening, Dad was watching a TV weather report. "Chicago's raining," he shouted.

"And where are you?" I asked, thinking that since he was in Florida, he didn't need to worry about the rain in Chicago.

"Kalamazoo, Michigan," he shouted back, naming one of the many college towns in which we had lived.

"Oh no!" My mind raced, trying to think about what to give him when he got disoriented. Was it an eighth of a teaspoon of salt in eight ounces of water or was it orange juice or ice cream or more nitro cream? I got up and started towards him but when I got in front of him I saw his grin.

"How about Clearwater, Florida."

That was my father's idea of a joke. I'd asked him where he was often enough. He was telling me to stop worrying...and to stop asking.

I got an excellent e-mail from my brother.

Dear Sis,

I am elated over your success with Dad's treatment. It sounds like something out of a movie. I only wish we had heard about this treatment when mother was alive. It seems like it might have helped her. Give Dad Sandi's and my love and tell him our every thought is with him. Ask him to call us when he has a chance.

Love, M.

My brother's support made me feel good.

23
No False Hope
Tuesday, October 17
Day Fifteen, Medication Day Twelve

Dad took the steps to Dr. Hammesfahr's Institute without a
pause. Behind him came a tall, thin man with a balding head,
who leapt up the stairs two at a time.

"You do a great job on the stairs!" I said. "How long
ago did you have your stroke?"

"Twenty-four years ago. I had a brain tumor. They
took it out, but nine days later I had a bleed. I've been like
this ever since." He indicated his clenched arm and tight fist.

Another story, another life, another potential
recovery. What a job the people at the Institute had! Every
day was a new start for another patient's recovery and they
already knew that the patient was going to get better.

Dad said hi to everyone and sat in his favorite red and
beige wing chair.

"How are you?" he asked a woman on the other side
of the room.

"Not too good," she said. "How are you?"

"I'm always good, except for the pain."

"I don't have any pain," she said.

"You're lucky." Sharon walked through the room on
her way to Summer's office. "There's the one who causes all

the pain." Dad pointed at Sharon the Shot Nurse and made sure he said it loud enough that she heard him.

"No pain, no gain!" Sharon whipped back, as she left the room. She always wore nurse's pajamas and her white nurse's coat over the top. Today's outfit was covered with tiny roses. She looked as though she'd walked out of a children's ward, bouncing around in her tennis shoes and her little flowers.

We saw Dr. Uzo in one of the downstairs rooms. She studied Dad's records. His blood pressure was 104/72. "Is that the correct reading?" she asked.

"I wrote it down. If that is what it says, that's it."

"We are not going to give you more magnesium today, no shot. And I'd like you to decrease your Accupril. In the morning, take only half a tablet. One more thing, I'd like you to drink four glasses of water with an eighth of a teaspoon of salt in each, every day for the next five days."

"Yech!" I said.

Dr. Uzo ignored me and continued. "It is part of the adjustments that we will be making this week to be sure that you are at your optimum level of medications. Don't worry about these changes. We want your blood vessels at their optimum levels."

Her badge read Nkem. I tried a few pronunciations in my mind. N-Kay-em, Nicky-em, Nick-em. "How do you pronounce your first name?" I asked as we were leaving.

"Kem," she said.

I tried Kemuzo as one word. It sounded like a mystic with powers far beyond the normal. It might have been a heroine in a movie. I wondered what it meant as she clicked away in her high heeled black pumps with the pearls and gold braid down the back.

Dad sang on the way to the motel,
"You're the cream in my coffee
You're the salt in my stew
You will always be

My necessity
I'd be lost without you."
"Wait until I put the salt in your drinking water. Then see if you think I'm your necessity," I teased him.
"I like salt water," Dad countered.
After lunch we headed to the Educational Session at the Clearwater Yacht Club. Diane Hartley, the physical therapist, was speaking when we got there. "Do exercises for a few minutes and then wait awhile to repeat them. If your physical therapist has questions, I will answer every one. Tell her to call. Sometimes I get behind, but I do get all the calls answered," she reassured everyone.
"Now I have to talk to you about sex. I don't know why I have to talk about it, especially alone. I'm the only woman in this threesome, and I have pale skin and when I blush everyone can see it. I think that the men ought to be in on this discussion, too. Don't you think so?"
There was a rousing "yes!" in response.
"Well, they're right outside. Would you please go and get them, Donna?" Through the windows we could all see Dr. Hammesfahr and Dr. Gimon on the boat dock, deep in conversation.
When they came inside, Diane demurred to Dr. Gimon, the psychologist. There was a handout, which he ignored.
"Making love can be accomplished in a variety of ways," he began. "There is more than one position. Be creative. Use the edge of the bed. Keep your sense of humor. Be sensitive to each other. You know each other better than anyone else in the world. And don't give up. If at first you don't succeed, try, try, again.
"Everyone wants to have a normal sex life. What is normal? You probably define normal as what you had before the stroke. But remember, making love does not have to be just intercourse. Caressing and kissing and affection are

needed, as well. Utilize all the functioning areas. It helps both of you become emotionally stronger. "A stroke is like an earthquake, quick and sudden. You have to adapt to that sudden change in your life. Talk about your feelings. Good verbal interaction is important. And of course, some of you may improve your sex life with all this trying."

Everyone laughed.

"The stroke affects the caregivers as well as the person who had the stroke," Dr. Gimon went on. "Most of you got here because you had a caregiver bring you here, but there is always some resentment and anger on the part of the caregiver. The caregiver says, 'He did this to me. He had this stroke. He made me responsible.' Remember, caregivers have a responsibility to themselves as well as to the stroke patient. If the caregiver gets tired or fatigued it contributes to depression in both caregiver and patient.

"Caregivers, it is not selfish of you to say, 'I need a break.' Patients, you make sure that they take that break, and you both will be much happier."

Donna raised her hand. "I told you last week that Dr. Hammesfahr was treating me for post-polio syndrome," she began. "Six months ago, I couldn't walk up stairs. I had to pull myself up with my arms, so I am much better now. But for the last month or so, I thought I hadn't had any change. I was moaning to myself about it as I walked my dog down the beach. I thought maybe this treatment was not going to work.

Finally, I turned around and began to walk back up the beach, and I saw my footprints. Instead of being duck-toed and far apart, they were in a straight line, like a normal person's feet would be. My gait and my balance were much better. I just hadn't noticed that things had changed." Her face crinkled up into her warm smile.

"I got depressed because I had not been observant enough, just as some of you may. Don't forget to observe yourself carefully. And caregivers should watch as well. You will get better and better, just like I am still getting better. Remember to look behind you and see where you have been."

This advice hung over the room as Dr. Hammesfahr began speaking. I left the table to get dad some fruit and cookies from the buffet. We already had our twenty-four-ounce bottles of water.

"I liked what Dr. Gimon said about hugs. Remember, it is much harder to hug someone in a wheel chair or a recliner. Families have to make an effort to provide the touching and hugging that are necessary. People can do without their sense of sight, hearing, smell or taste, but they *cannot* survive without being touched. A good way to do that is to massage the sore muscles or muscles that have not been actively used for a while. Families are vital to a patient's recovery.

"The patient wants to be valued as a human with much experience and knowledge. They want to be important and useful. They want someone to care when they hurt or cheer them up when they feel down. Playing games, watching a TV show with them, talking about your problems as well as theirs makes them feel that they are still part of a family. Don't exclude them.

"Often stroke patients are no longer able to do things for themselves. Things that they loved to do, like play golf, or go to the store, or drive a car are impossible. They can't do simple things like fasten a bra or open a door or brush their teeth. Patients can't zip their pants or button their shirts. Getting a cup of coffee, moving out of a chair or responding to a question requires major effort. Their bodies don't work well and they are full of pain. They get frustrated and this can lead to becoming sedentary and disillusioned. Television can become their sole outreach to the world.

"As a result of all of these problems, some of you come here fighting depression. This depression creates stress, which makes your muscles contract even more. The pain worsens and that makes for more depression. If you have had no improvement in many years you tend to think that you will never improve.

Stroke patients have notoriously low self-esteem. They think that they are not worth the time, money or effort it would take to get the therapy. They often can't or won't make the decision to come for therapy, so caregivers, you have to make the choice about when to come for therapy, and it is not easy.

"Caregivers get stuck in their situation. Often they are overburdened and have little outside help. They continue to do the overwhelming job of caring for their loved ones, but don't have energy left over to seek new solutions for their problems. They are meeting the emotional and physical needs of the patient, but no one is helping them with their own emotional needs and physical exhaustion. All this is exacerbated by the fear that whatever they do might make their loved ones worse and that it would be their fault.

"While depression is a symptom of the disease of stroke, it also affects the caregivers and they lose hope, as well. In addition to the depression, caregivers often feel guilty. They feel guilty about their frustration at losing their own freedom. They think that they could have done something differently and the stroke might not have occurred. They think that if they had been able to decrease the stress on the patient that the stroke might not have occurred. They wonder, "Why me?" or "Why us?"

"They feel anger, too. Sometimes it is anger because they are now required to spend all of their time caring for demanding invalids or anger that the stroke victim didn't take better care. They also fear that another stroke would occur while they are in charge and it would be their fault. They are afraid, worse yet, that they might have a stroke and no longer be able to care for their charges.

"Added to that is the fear of trying something new, something that might make their life or the life of their loved ones worse. They know how to manage extremely difficult situations, but any change is difficult and frightening. They lose hope that their world can ever change except, possibly, to worsen."

Dr. Hammesfahr certainly could go into depth about topics he cared about. His lectures were perceptive and insightful. Of course, this was the educational session. What did I expect?

"Spiritual beliefs are often ignored by the medical profession," Dr. Hammesfahr went on, "but they play a big part in the attitude of patients towards their recovery. Recovery is dramatically a mental, physical *and* spiritual process. The patients are changed spiritually, and so are their families.

It is interesting to note that many patients who have returned with family do not wish that the stroke had never happened because of the increased closeness and strength that they achieved as a result of the stroke. Except for small children with strokes, the families report that they have reconnected in what some call their 'Golden Moments,' during this time. When they get to the Institute and they see themselves recovering, joy and hope fill their hearts and families are drawn even closer together.

"Are there any questions?" Dr. Hammesfahr pointed to one of the up-stretched hands and called on a svelte woman who looked about fifty.

"I'm gaining weight since I started taking Accupril. I've been the same weight since I was twenty and now I've put on five pounds."

"There are some problems with taking Accupril. People report that they have a tendency to gain weight, and it doesn't do much for your libido. Those of you who are just starting to take it watch your diet now, at the beginning. Try three days on a diet and one day off. That has seemed to work for some of our patients."

Question after question was shot up to the front of the room. Dr. Hammesfahr answered them all, smoothly inserting his own agenda for the day into the answers.

"You will need less medicine as you go along. Two or three years down the road you may need only a third to half the medicine you take now. You will not be on the same dosage for the rest of your life. The dose is important. Lipitor dilates the vessels in small doses, but constricts them in large doses. You may even change medications if these don't work for you. We give the ultrasound three to six months to become normal then the arteries should start to heal. The end result should be stable, healthy arteries."

The session continued, with lots of questions flying back and forth across the room at a very fast pace.

"My leg feels like it's going to buckle. Why?" asked a patient with a walker.

"Don't give up your walker just yet," Diane answered. "These are new muscles you are using and they are not strong yet. First the movement comes back, but your balance will take much longer. We don't want you falling in the meantime. When you're sitting down, raise your knee up and push down on it with your hands. That will strengthen it."

"My arm muscles seem more relaxed, but I still can't move my hand," said a woman from her wheelchair.

"Remember, your hand has been clenched for a long time." Diane said. "You need to stretch the ligaments out manually. Try pushing your fingers back with your good hand." She demonstrated. "If you can't get your hand open, try twisting the thumb. It will open right up." She used this technique and immediately the woman's fingers loosened to a gentle curl. "See! It always works."

A fireman asked about carbon monoxide poisoning.

"We've treated drowning, strangulation, all kinds of hypoxic episodes, where the patient was robbed of oxygen," Dr. Hammesfahr said.

Suddenly, I realized that he was talking about incidents like the one that Heather experienced in her accident. She had been without oxygen.

"The results are pretty good with these patients. It works a little differently from the way it does with a stroke patient, who may have a significant improvement in the first three weeks. These patients tend to start recovery slowly and speed up as they go along."

After the meeting broke up, Debbie, the woman who had first answered my questions when I called the Institute, came over to us. My father had told her about my friends, Brooks, Dorothy, and Heather. She encouraged me to bring them to an Educational Session.

"But they are not sure," I said. "Heather might get depressed or angry instead of better."

"But she could have major recovery. We've seen some with ninety percent recovery," Debbie said. "How could they deny their child that opportunity?"

"A ninety percent recovery? For Heather?"

I called my friends as soon as we got back to the motel, and told them about the discussion that day.

"Every person we speak to has some relative or friend who would benefit from this treatment," Dorothy said. "We will come, but we're not going to bring Heather. It would be too difficult for us to keep her moving so her circulation doesn't get cut off. I don't want her having seizures while we're trying to listen. The problem is we don't have an afternoon nurse right now. I'm going to try to get the morning nurse to stay longer. I'll call you tomorrow after I talk with her. Maybe we could meet for lunch before the Educational Session."

"Great. I'll find a place."

"There is no such thing as false hope," Dorothy said. "It's a sign on the wall in Heather's room. I really believe it." I knew that there was also no such thing as a little hope. It was like being a little pregnant. Either you had hope or you didn't. I wanted their hope to bulge inside their hearts. I wanted hope to consume them until their conversation could no longer be about anything but their hope for Heather. I wanted them to have enough hope to come on Thursday and listen and find out if this treatment would work for Heather.

I imagined Heather's glowing face looking up at Dad and me, her eyes sparkling. If an angel had touched anyone, it was Heather. If anyone deserved a miracle, it was she.

24
So Much Work
Wednesday, October 18
Day Sixteen, Medication Day Thirteen

"Sling-a-ling, sling-a ling, ding-a-ling" the teacher on the other side of the waiting room sang out. "That's what the dyslexic kids called the program I taught. It was modeled after a program to treat stroke victims. I wasn't surprised to hear that this therapy works with dyslexic children." The teacher, Rebecca, had taught elementary school and had a non-stop monologue on the subject, but she was pretty interesting if you had ever taught special education students. I had, and I listened avidly.

"Dirk and Nancy walked through. "Look what he can do! He can hold the water bottle in his bad hand." Nancy was elated.

Dirk demonstrated his new prowess by shifting his water bottle from his right hand back to his left hand. "Fishing pole, too," he said, adding another short sentence to his repertoire.

We were taken in to see Debbie, who was going to check Dad's ultrasound for the third time. She got Dad settled in the big wing chair.

"How long have you worked here?" I asked her.

"I got this job two days after I finished school, a year and a half ago. Everybody in the office interviewed me.

They called me the next morning and asked me to come to work for them that day. This office was too far away from home and they offered too little money, but I said yes, though I told them I couldn't start until the following Monday. I've been here ever since."

Dad started teasing her, parodying "You Made Me Love You."

"I drive you crazy,
I didn't want to do it,
And everybody knew it."

She laughed, but then she always had a cheery outlook.

I watched the screen as Dad's right side came up. The picture didn't look much different from the one taken the week before. There was still a strong upsweep, but it had a little bend at the top. The down sweep was long and jagged. The same was true for his left side but it was much lower in height.

"With low blood pressure, it takes much longer for the ultrasound to turn around," Debbie said. "It could be three to six months until we see some change."

For him, the optimum meter per second flow of blood was .26. Dad's was .52 and .64. That sounded like a long way from .26.

"This is where the therapy becomes customized," Debbie said. "Wait for the doctor."

Dr. Webber explained that because Dad had low blood pressure, he would have to wait for the medicine to build up in his system in order to see a change in the ultrasound. It might take a long time. With high blood pressure, the arteries open right up.

"This is so much work," Dad sighed, as we left the office. His shoulders sank and he walked slowly to the car. I waited while he laboriously slammed the door and struggled to fasten the seat belt. He sang, but it was a sad song.

"I ain't got no body,

And nobody cares for me."
I'm so sad and lonely,
Won't somebody come and take a chance on me."
    The phone was ringing when we got to the motel. It was Brooks. "We're going to come down for the Educational Session tomorrow. We got the morning nurse to agree to stay for the afternoon."
    "Great. The session starts at two-thirty."
    "We thought we'd come for lunch."
    "I've been wanting to go to this restaurant, Leverocks, that's right near the Yacht Club. It's a fish place on the water. The views will be great." I gave them the directions and arranged the meeting time. "I am so happy you are coming," I said.
    "Wipe that silly grin off your face," Dad chided. "You look like you swallowed the canary."
    "While we're down here, it's a parrot," I said, thinking of the flock of green ones we often saw flying over the bay. "Brooks and Dorothy are coming on Thursday. I am so pleased. I want them to understand what Dr. Hammesfahr is doing. Once they understand they will have a hard time saying no to Heather's treatment."
    "You're so sure that it will work."
    "What do you think?
    "I think it will work. But it's hard work. It is going to be hard for them as well as for Heather. They may not want to do it. Just because you think they ought to do it doesn't make them want to undertake it."
    "They're retired," I said. "They might as well do this. Anyway, we are all going to have a great fish lunch at a beautiful restaurant!"
    "Good start," Dad said.

25
White Lightening
Thursday, October 19
Day Seventeen, Medication Day Fourteen

"Robin, I feel rotten this morning. All yucky."
Dad was sitting in his usual chair watching TV when I got up. My first activity every morning was to take his blood pressure. I got out the digital machine and strapped it around his arm. I move slowly in the morning so it was easy for me to simply stand and look at the numbers rolling through the machine. Dad was not walking well either.

His blood pressure was 104/62. I didn't know how he could move with blood pressure so low. I did as I'd been told, and gave him eighth teaspoon of salt in eight ounces of water. I wondered if they would change his medicine again. We were getting close to the end of our stay and I worried that his medications would not be settled by the time we went home. That would leave a mess for my sister to handle. It would be difficult enough for her, since she had not been down here with him to sit through all of the Education Sessions. I waited ten minutes. When I took Dad's blood pressure again it was 116/68. That was almost within his range.

I was amazed. It was so simple. If his blood pressure was down, it reacted immediately to salt. All he had to do to keep it up was eat a little salt. When it was higher he felt much better and could walk more easily. This was a magnificent discovery! It allowed him to keep his blood pressure within his range by himself. He could tell when he was getting sluggish, and pop a salt fix. It acted like white lightening.

Dr. Webber took his blood pressure again when we got to the Institute. It was 119/73. I told him about this morning's low reading. "Are you drinking your sixty-four ounces of water?" he asked Dad.

We both nodded.

"Take his blood pressure when he has a setback, and again when he is feeling especially strong. That will help him gage his optimum blood pressure. He shouldn't worry about it unless it is out of range for two days, sooner if there are symptoms like you found this morning. Accupril has the biggest effect on blood pressure. Cut his Accupril in the morning. Don't give him any until lunch." He wrote out the new schedule, 0-1-1-3.

Before we left, I asked my usual list of questions. "What is 'nitro as needed? How long does it take for magnesium to build up in Dad's system?"

When we left the office, Ellen, the young blonde girl, was walking in with her mother. "Ellen, you are walking so well," I blurted. "You aren't even limping."

"Yeah," she said. "It happened this morning. I'm walking much better. Mom and I took a long walk this morning."

"Did you reward yourselves?"

"With pancakes. I even cut them myself." She pointed to her stricken arm now hanging loosely by her side.

"I bet you're so happy!" The glow on her face left no doubt.

"We are leaving tomorrow," she said. "Are you going to be at the meeting this afternoon?"

"Of course. We wouldn't miss it."

"Good. I want to get your e-mail address and take a picture of you and your Dad."

Sharon whizzed by. "That salt has improved your disposition," she commented to Dad.

"Am I that wide open?" he asked.

"I can read you like a book," was her departing shot. There was a wide grin on Dad's face.

The door swung open and a nurse wheeled her patient, Fanny, into the room. Fanny's previously rigid body was now nestled in her chair. She once had such spastic paralysis in her tongue and mouth that her face was a distorted mask. Now, I thought she might have been smiling.

"She's a lot better," I said to her nurse.

"Yes, she's much better. Her body is beginning to loosen up."

Again, the attitudes and the positive changes in this place swelled our hearts. Even Fanny could get better.

Leverocks was located next to the bridge that led to Sand Key. It had a spectacular view of the currents and eddies making ripples on the water. Small fishing boats, tourist boats and para-sailers passed each other going in and out. There were a few sunbathers on the beach and two brave souls were splashing at the water's edge.

We were seated next to another stroke victim. He was not someone I had seen at the Institute, just one of the many in Florida. Their wheelchairs and walkers were everywhere on city streets and in suburban malls. They became part of the landscape, a barely noticed group of bent bodies that the rest of us brushed by without seeing. These were people who were left in nursing homes and visited on weekends by obligated children. Like the people in Dad's retirement hotel, they were roused for meals or when the staff provided a little entertainment. They didn't instigate new activities for themselves and no one was capable of entertaining them all the time. Not even their memories kept them amused. They sat in their armchairs in the lobby and faded into subconscious thought. We had the opportunity to change all that by handing them a phone number.

"Do you suppose that when you go home, people in your retirement home who have strokes will want to come here and get well?" I asked Dad.

He shook his head. "No. I don't think I would have come if I had seen it in the magazine. I needed you to push me a bit. You get to the point where you try so hard to walk or to use your hand and you can't do it. Pretty soon you give up. There was no hope that I was ever going to get any better. If I had seen that ad in the magazine I would have thought yeah-h-h, and not done anything about it. I think when you're discouraged it takes someone with a lot of oomph to get you started again, especially with something like this."

"Don't you think that people will want to come when they see the changes in you?"

"I don't think they will see the changes in me."

"You may be right, as strange as it seems. People are not very observant about themselves, so I guess they might be even less observant about you."

"They need someone to help them. Old people who have strokes are so down on themselves they won't initiate anything. Look at the people at the clinic. Almost all have someone to guide them, to invigorate them and say, 'Come on, you can do this.' Unless people have someone who will encourage them, they won't come. Someone else has to make the decision for them. Someone else must push them to try one more time."

"I will be interested in whether anyone chooses to come to the Institute. Let me know. What about that cute woman who has lunch with you, Theadora? Why is she so spacey?"

"I don't know. She remembers a lot of things about her house in Arizona and her friends back there. Then suddenly she says, 'I don't remember any more,' and stops talking. She has hardening of the arteries."

"You know, maybe it's those arteries that feed the part of the brain that controls balance, memory, vision, and concentration. Maybe if those arteries were opened up a little and more blood got to her brain, she would remember better."

"I should bring her down here with me," said Dad, ever eager to be a hero to a pretty woman.

"Not you, Daddy. Her children will have to bring her down here. Don't they have a home in Tampa?"

"There's not a thing wrong with her physically. It's just her memory." He began to stand up. "I have to go to the bathroom," he said, ending that conversation. He limped off toward the back of the restaurant.

The people at the next table ordered some non-alcoholic beer. I remembered that stuff from college when I was too young to drink. We called it Near Beer. What a great idea! Our family had always loved the time of day when the sun sets and we sat down together and talked about our day's activities and concerns. But cocktail hour without the cocktails didn't work. I kept jumping up to do things. Dad and I sat with long pauses. We got restless. I would read the newspaper. Dad would float off into thought. But add a bottle of beer and a glass of wine, and conversation flowed. The pleasures of our daily rituals would be restored. Our pattern of life could return to normal, defined by what it was before the stroke. I called the waitress over and ordered a bottle for Dad.

He came back to the table a few minutes later. "Do I have a surprise for you." I wiggled my shoulders, hardly able to sit in my seat. The waitress brought Dad a cold beer with an iced mug to pour it in.

"What's this? You're going to let me drink this?"

"It's non-alcoholic! Taste it!"

He poured a little in the mug and brought it to his lips. "Fantastic. It tastes just like beer. Can I have as much as I want?"

"As long as you're paying for it. Live it up."

He reached over for the saltshaker and salted his beer. "Life is good."

"You are going to be so revved up on that salt you won't be able to sit still during the meeting this afternoon."

Our friends Brooks and Dorothy arrived and joined us at the table.

"How are you doing, Woody?" asked Dorothy.

"I can really taste this beer. I haven't been able to taste anything for years. I think my sense of taste is coming back."

I was amazed. Just a month earlier he would have said, "Ecch, I can't tell. Everything tastes the same to me."

"That's a wonderful thing." Dorothy looked over the menu. We ordered and the waitress brought our salads. The topic of conversation immediately turned to the Institute.

"We saw a videotape of Dr. Hammesfahr on TV. It was a repeat of an NBC program from six months ago. They talked to a patient who had recovered his speech. He had a slow, halting, raspy voice on the program. Then we met this man, the one on TV, yesterday. I didn't recognize him. His face is different. His whole bearing is different and his speech is really good," I said.

"I assume that by 'different' you mean better." Dorothy put the menu down to listen.

"Yes, much better. Much, much, better. Of course, this is six months after the TV program. He has had six months more of recovery. The same thing could happen to Heather."

"We couldn't bring her along," Brooks said. "She has to be turned every two hours or her circulation gets cut off."

"But she's very alert," Dorothy said. "She watches 'All My Children' and laughs at all the innuendoes. She likes dirty jokes, too. We always tell the nurses to remember that she is a thirty-four year old woman, not a child."

The waitress brought our main courses as Dorothy continued. "People love to work with Heather. When we were involved in the patterning we had to have dozens of volunteers move her body. Literally hundreds of people worked with her over the years. A woman who did acupuncture on pets, a veterinarian, was one of our patterners. She introduced us to Lily Tomlin, who came to work with Heather once and invited us to her show. Afterwards, in her dressing room, she perched herself on the wheelchair and put her arm around Heather. After that, we always called Heather's left leg her 'Lily Leg.' She sent Heather little presents from her shows for a long time. She even donated money in Heather's name to the street people in LA. All kinds of people love Heather. But we finally gave up on the patterning when Heather stopped getting any better."

"I'm glad you decided to come and find out about this treatment," I said. "Heather is so charismatic."

"We don't want to change that. If these medications made her unhappy or depressed I don't know what we'd do."

"You'd do the same things that other parents of depressed children do," Dad said, using his deep, reassuring counseling voice.

"Didn't you say she was always a happy child?" I asked.

"Yes. She was before the accident." Dorothy sighed and sat quietly, remembering. "It would be wonderful to see her improve and then have a huge party in Chicago for all the people who helped with her patterning behavior all those years," Dorothy mused.

"Except we don't have an apartment there any more," Brooks said.

"But I do," I offered. "I would be delighted to host that kind of a party as long as it's in the summer. We're not going to spend any more winters in Chicago. But what a great party that would be!"

There it was. Hope. When you hope, the first thing that happens is you plan. You start thinking, about people who care for your father or daughter and would like to see the changes in them. Who would understand what this means? Who would share the joy?

"I guess we shouldn't plan a party before Heather improves," Dorothy said. "We don't know if it will work for her, yet."

We all tried to come down a little as we left the restaurant for the three-block drive to the Yacht Club. The Education Session was at the back, near the boat docks. We sat at the tables outside, waiting for the catering people to finish setting up the goodies for the meeting. They hauled in a large iced pan full of water bottles.

"How do you feel?" I asked Brooks.

"Anticipatory, excited, reflective, nervous, like a yo-yo," he said. "How old are you, Woody?"

"Eighty-three," Dad said.

"Eighty-two," I corrected him.

"You better watch her," Dorothy said. "She's giving away your age."

"Let her. She can give away all the years she wants." Dad got the giggles as he made the joke. He was hyper, like a young boy who has had his first illicit taste of alcohol. I knew that that beer was non-alcoholic. The salt must have sent him. I wondered what his blood pressure was right now. I bet it was high.

The meeting began with the usual introductions of everyone in attendance. At first, I'd thought that was a little hokey but I didn't any more. It set a tone for the meeting. It established that it was all right to talk and ask questions. It also gave patients who'd had a breakthrough an opportunity to describe their accomplishments and to encourage the rest of us to look for these small changes. Donna addressed each patient by name and asked where he or she was from. People were there from England and Germany and France as well as California, Ohio, Connecticut, and of course, Florida.

Donna asked them about the changes they had observed. Patients reported such improvements as being able to touch their thumbs and their first fingers together.

Sometimes they choked up with emotion when they talked. "I hope I get better and better."

Sometimes they reported progress. "My wife's personality is back to when she was a teenager."

Sometimes, big changes occurred. "Her walk, vision, and speech are normal."

Sometimes, small ones. "Her finger on her frozen arm moved."

Sometimes they expressed their thanks. "Dr. Hammesfahr, I hope you are not homophobic because if this works I'm going to plant a big kiss on your cheek!"

Sometimes they offered services. "I'll do a web site." Everyone wanted a letter-writing campaign to Medicare to reestablish the treatment as an approved Medicare expense. Patients wanted all stroke victims to have access to this treatment, not just the wealthy.

Sometimes they told stories about how the stroke had affected their lives. Dan was a middle school teacher in California who taught in a gang-infested neighborhood. He'd had his stroke two days before being named Cable Using Teacher of the Year. He was going to speak in front of Congress. When he finally went back to teaching, his students rallied around him. He couldn't use his left arm and his left leg was weak. He got tired easily. But students fought for the privilege of pushing his wheelchair from classroom to classroom.

"I couldn't do anything but work hard at getting better," Dan said. "All of the students were watching me as a role model. One day I was giving a test, when I noticed that Selema, a girl in the front row, was struggling.

"'Is it hard?' I asked her.

"'Just because something is hard, or because it is not something I really want to do, or because it is painful, these are not reasons to quit,' she said.

"Where did you learn that? I asked.

"'You taught me,' she said.

"I could not have taught her that lesson if I had not had my stroke. Selema's ambition is to be a teacher. I don't know whether my response to my stroke was a good influence or not, but I know that I can't let my students down. I have to keep trying to get better."

No wonder this man was an award-winning teacher.

No one at these sessions ever talked down to the patients. They listened, even if patients had a hard time or took awhile to find the words or get them through their tangled tongues. They did not ignore the patients and talk only to the caregivers, or speak to patients as if they were somehow more childish as a result of paralysis. That habit in other doctors and nurses always drove my father crazy.

Joe, an artist who had first been treated at the Institute two years ago, began to tell us about the exercises he used while recovering. I liked the deep breathing one because it felt like a Cosmic Sigh. I also liked the idea of tricking the brain by exercising the good arm first and then the bad arm, then exercising both of them. The brain thought the bad arm was an extension of the good one, and that made the bad one work better. Weird, but true.

The questions started coming for Dr. Hammesfahr. "Do hearing and sight return?"

"In your case, probably," he said. "They come back. Most anything that works at all will work better. If it doesn't work at all before we start, then it's more of a crap shoot whether it will come back or not."

Dr. Hammesfahr sounded knowledgeable, secure, relaxed. I knew, because I had listened to several of these question and answer sessions that appeared not to have an agenda, that he most certainly did have one. He made his points as the questions came rolling in. Complaints, or maybe pleas for help, tinkled like xylophone notes across the room.

"I'm so cold all the time."

"My joints ache."

"I'm so tired."

"How about smoking?"

Dr. Hammesfahr paused before he issued this ominous statement. "Smoking affects your blood pressure a lot. You can see it dramatically constrict blood vessels on the ultrasound. We had a patient a few years back. We could *not* get control of the opening and closing of his blood vessels. We'd give him medications and wait twenty minutes to retest. The test would be worse. Finally, one of the staff saw him go outside on the front porch and smoke a cigarette while he was waiting for the next test. An artery can change from eighty percent open to twenty percent open, maybe less, within fifteen minutes of smoking a cigarette. We actually documented this on the ultrasound. Don't even think about smoking."

I thought about Dad's sixty years of smoking prior to his stroke. He must have been a strong person; it took a long time before he had a stroke as a result of it.

"What about patterning?" Brooks asked. He and Dorothy and a host of volunteers worked on patterning with Heather for seven years. She was one of the few adult patients who had tried that method of recovery. Most were children.

"The problem with patterning," Dr. Hammesfahr said, "is that in order for it to work the brain must work better. When that happens then patterning works, but if we can make the brain work better you may have no need for patterning at all."

"Why do we have to drink so much water?"

"You must drink enough water to allow you to take enough medicine to heal. Drink your water. If you don't drink your water, you won't get better."

"In what order do things usually return?"

"There are no guarantees and everyone is different. But generally, personality, spirits, energy, and memory come back first, then the legs, feet, arms, and hands in that order. Things that are controlled by both sides of the brain, like swallowing and balance seem to come back faster because both sides improve. Nitro seems to work on the outer ring," he continued, referring to the concentric circle chart we saw on the videotape when we first came to the Institute.

"How many patients in this room were depressed or taking antidepressants as a result of their stroke before coming here?" he asked. All of the patient's hands shot up. "And how many caregivers and spouses were depressed or on antidepressants?" Eighty percent of the hands rose.

"This is a family disease. It affects everyone in the family. Lots of people call it 'our stroke'"

"Why don't other doctors do this?"

"It is not as easy as it looks. We have a lot of expensive equipment. The doctors must change the way that they treat patients, seeing them every day devoting a large amount of time to them. They can't do it with a fifteen minute appointment. Our doctors are very sophisticated people. They see a patient's charts every day. Finally, there is no money to be made in it. Right now, Medicare won't pay for it. Some universities have sent physicians here to learn about it, but they have to go through a lot of hoops to do it.

"This treatment is preventive as well as curative," Dr. Hammesfahr went on. "Not one of the people we have treated in the last five years who stayed with the therapy has had another stroke. That is an unusually positive statistic. National statistics show that forty percent of stroke victims have a second stroke within five years, and thirty percent have one within three years of their last stroke. But of the

thousands of patients who have come to the Institute and stayed with the therapy, not one has had a stroke since.
"I want to point out that Dr. Robinson has been keeping meticulous records of his blood pressure readings. Because of that, we were able to pinpoint his ideal blood pressure very easily. I urge all of you to do the same. If you come in here with detailed records of your blood pressure and how you felt when it was taken, it would be a great help to us."

Dr. Hammesfahr walked over to Dad's chair when he said that. These sessions made everyone happy, but those praise-filled remarks made Dad feel like a sixth grader who has been rewarded with a star for perfect schoolwork.

The meeting broke up on that positive note. Brooks and Dorothy headed over to Dr. Hammesfahr. They talked intently for about fifteen minutes. Finally, they joined Dad and me at one of the outside tables.

"What did he say?" I asked.

"He said that he thought he could help. We have to do this, Robin. We couldn't deny Heather this opportunity." Dorothy was adamant now.

"If you had three goals for Heather what would they be?" Dad asked.

"The relaxation of her muscles, so her spasms would decrease. Second, that she could swallow. Third, that she could hold her head up."

"Isn't there some far out dream of improvement that you want? Dream big," I encouraged her.

"I'm waiting for, 'Hi mom!'"

"I don't think that is too much to ask. There is a chance. She vocalizes. Now all she has to do is to get her teeth, tongue, lips, and mind to work as one. You know she can think. She just needs to verbalize her thoughts."

"I have another saying hung in Heather's room, besides the one about no false hope: A realist, in our time, is one who believes in miracles."

"This treatment looks like a miracle," I said, "but it is just very creative thinking by a very smart doctor. Of course, creative thinking is a miracle in itself."

We walked silently and slowly towards the cars, keeping pace with Dad and his cane. "Call me before you go," Dorothy said, as she hugged me good-by.

"I might not be able to. The last few days will be very hectic. I'll call you as soon as I get home, okay?"

Brooks was waiting for me on the other side of the car. He put both arms around me. "I can't thank you enough," he whispered. His voice broke in the middle of the words. I climbed into the car and closed the door.

"You did good." Dad smiled at me.

"Now that they have caught Hope, they won't be able to get over it." I teased.

"I guess they will just have to suffer, suffer, suffer, with it."

"I don't feel bad at all. In fact I feel pretty good about what we've just accomplished."

When we got to the motel, the phone was ringing. It was my sister. She was full of good cheer from her brief but restful northern vacation with her husband. I told her our good news, listing all of Dad's improvements over the past few days. Dad asked about his deposit to the bank. She promised to check on it. I was glad he had someone who loved him to look after him when he got home.

26
Dink Water/Don't Smoke
Friday, October 20
Day Eighteen, Medication Day Fifteen

Dad's blood pressure had been low again the previous night, 104/60. He was tired and he had a lot of pain in his arm. I gave him eight ounces of salt water and put a hot Epsom Salted towel on his arm. His blood pressure went up to 120/60 in ten minutes and his pain went away. White Lightening! It worked again. In the morning his arm was looser and his blood pressure was almost on target at 121/78. I put up DINK WATER on with the magnetic letters on the refrigerator.

Fanny was in the waiting room when we arrived. Her tongue was no longer protruding from her mouth.

"Is she smiling again?" I asked, looking at her beaming face.

"No, she's mad because I've just wiped her face," her nurse said. But she is much better. She's not stiff as a board anymore."

Summer rushed by, pausing long enough to give Dad a big hug. She was confident and smiling, a different girl from the one we'd met a few weeks ago. Sharon, in sneakers and her white nurse's outfit with the little pink roses, looked innocent enough, but she had two sharp needles in her hand ready to give Dad his magnesium shots. She was Sharon the Shot Nurse today.

"Let me show you how to do this," she said. It was the second time she had tried to get me to give Dad a shot. This time she indicated that I was to take the needles. "You'll have to do it when you get home."

"Oh no," I protested. "His doctor will do it, or my sister will have to learn how." But she ignored my protests as she cleaned my hands and Dad's skin. I took the needles and jabbed them into the soft fleshy skin below his waist.

"I always knew you were a pain in the rear end," he quipped. "Ever since you were a little girl."

"You can wait in the office for the doctor," Sharon indicated the room where we had first been interviewed.

This was our checkout appointment. Dad had to take off his shoes again, but he had stopped wearing those pesky socks weeks ago, so it was a lot easier.

Dr. Uzo sat down at the desk and began looking through Dad's records. "Sharon," she called. Sharon popped her head into the room. "Where are Dr. Robinson's blood pressure sheets?"

Sharon whipped into the office and opened Dad's medical file to the back. "I stapled them both to the back page where I keep my records. I'm sorry." She fixed the page and looked at Dad mischievously. "You always get me in trouble," she said. Then she hugged him. He just grinned.

Dr. Uzo began running through the same set of tests that had been done on the second day. She touched his feet and hands to see if he could feel the tiny metal prong. She ran it down the side of his face.

"How come I can feel my face better than I can feel my leg?" Dad asked.

"Your facial nerves come directly from the brain. Those nerves have a faster recovery than your arm and leg because they come through the spine," Dr. Uzo explained.

"I have my peripheral vision back," Dad said. "I can see all the way over to the right side." She tested him with a small rod and it was true. "Now I won't miss cards over there on the far right side when I play bridge."

Dr. Uzo began making a list of his Activities Of Daily Living (AODL) improvements. I wrote notes furiously.

Takes shower himself, gets in and out of the tub with better balance

Can dry his own back

Walks faster and with better gait

Arm has loosened up, hangs by his side

Thinks better

Words come more easily

Engages in word play

Hits his mouth more frequently with his food

Does not dribble out of the right side of his mouth as much

Can cross his legs (don't do it)

Peripheral vision returned

"We will give you a duplicate copy of the set of directions for your physician and the nursing home next week before you leave," Dr. Uzo said. "We will FAX the original copy to your doctor and to your nursing home. We will also give you a prescription for magnesium shots."

We nodded dutifully.

"I want you to keep a list of all of your improvements. If you don't, you will forget how much better you are getting. If you do, you will remember when things begin to happen. If you begin to get recovery, even a little bit, that area will keep improving. I want you to be observant and notice when these small changes take place."

"Now I'm just wondering," Dad said, "if the holes that they drilled in my head caused this stroke, because I didn't have any of the symptoms for a stroke. I didn't have high blood pressure and I didn't have high cholesterol."

"No, that couldn't have done it," Dr. Uzo said firmly.

"Dad, we've talked about this before. You had the stroke before they drilled the holes in your head. They drilled the holes because of the bleeding inside your skull. You had a stroke because you smoked for sixty years."

"Oh, that's not true," he protested.

"Dr. Uzo, please explain it to him."

"Your body can repair your lungs by itself, but you cannot repair your constricted blood vessels by yourself. The smoking caused the constricted blood vessels. It will take the medication a long time to repair the blood vessels. If you smoked for sixty years, don't expect that damage to disappear in a few months."

Dad didn't look happy about that. Our drive to the motel was quiet.

Finally, Dad said, "I still don't know why I had this stroke. I didn't have high blood pressure or cholesterol."

"You smoked for sixty years. Your blood vessels got constricted and damaged. That's what the doctor said this morning."

"I didn't hear her say that."

"She did." But he did not remember what he did not want to know in the first place.

We headed off to our afternoon appointment with Timothy at the educational psychologist's office. He repeated the tests he had done with Dad at our first appointment. He asked Dad the year, the month, the date, and the day. Then he brought out the tapping machine. This time, with his bad hand, Dad managed to push the metal bar down seven times in a minute. Last time, he could not hold his hand still enough to get his finger to touch the metal bar. He'd had a score of zero. Amazingly, with his left hand, his good hand, his score improved from forty-six taps a minute to sixty-five taps a minute. Everything that worked got better.

We went through the "What's Missing from This Picture" test, the decoding and organization tests, the concentration and short-term memory test, and the processing of words. It was interesting that when Dad was asked to give words that started with f, a, and s, I expected that he would use nouns as they were the easiest words, like fan, apple or sack, but Dad used words that were more complicated and abstract, like fantastic, anxious, and similar. When he defined words I noticed that he sometimes gave a second definition, such as for the word "sentence." He said it was time in jail or a series of words that made sense. Another one was "matchless," which he defined as a guy without a match. Then he laughed at his own joke and then redefined it as having no equal. He remembered the language of the test that he knew so well, and used that answer. Over and over he gave sophisticated answers that used the word play we so often engaged in as a family. Around our dining room table, whole conversations could be carried on while punning on a single word, all of us reveling in each new outrageous alteration of the original word.

After we finished, Timothy summarized his findings. "You have improvement in the following areas: Organization of Thoughts, Processing Information, Motor Skills, and Attention. You are more alert and energetic. What do you think?"

"I think the testing will do the Institute more good than me," Dad cracked.

"Pretty subtle," Timothy said.

"I came down here with the hopes of getting better."

"Both your mind and your physical actions are better." We both stood to leave. "You have a nice weekend."

"Did you bring your writing?" I asked.

"No I forgot," Timothy fidgeted.

"Keep working on it," I advised. "It will take courage for you to show it to others, but you have a story to tell and you need to tell it."

We climbed into our little green-mobile and began the trek down the wide streets toward our temporary home.

"That didn't seem like much," Dad sighed.

"Dad, a little improvement means that you will keep getting better and better in that area. You will get better physically and better mentally, too."

"I want it to be all of a sudden. I want it to be faster."

"That's not going to happen. It will be little by little. Think about how great it will be as you go though the months seeing more and more changes."

"I'd still like to see all the changes at once. I could look back on them with as much pleasure as I anticipate them." He paused. "What if your sister doesn't see any difference when I get home?"

"Do you have as much pain?"

"No."

"Tell her that the pain is gone. She's not supposed to be able to see that." I sensed my answer was too quick and flippant. He was worried about the rest of the world, not just our little Clearwater cocoon. "Just the fact that you can take a shower by yourself will be a big difference. Shave, every day. Brush your teeth with the electric toothbrush. Believe me, she will notice."

"No one at the Fort Armstrong will notice."

"What do they notice now?"

"Not much."

"Then they won't notice much when you go back. Being observant is not a talent everyone has."

We drank water the rest of the way home, knowing that we would be near a toilet for the rest of the evening. It is quite easy to drink twenty-four ounces of water in a few minutes once you get used to it.

27
Playing Angels
Saturday, October 21
Day Nineteen, Medicine Day Sixteen

There was a large white heron standing in the shallows of the bay when we took our morning walk. It was perfectly still, looking down into the water. Its beady yellow eyes never moved from the spot it had staked out. Its long black legs were rigid. Its skinny black beak was waiting. That kind of focus on a project is rare in humans, but we had been as focused as possible on this therapy for almost three weeks.

Now, our focus on Dad's illness was coming to a close. The day seemed the same as any other but there was something else happening. It was as subtle as a change in the breeze. Dad took his blood pressure. It was 127/76. Right on target for him. We ate breakfast, took a walk, and watched the talking heads on TV, but it was different now. It was not as exciting. Not as thrilling. There was not as much expectation. There was more repetitive work. Dad was entering the next phase of recovery. He was going to have to make permanent the lifestyle changes he had been practicing in Clearwater. We would take our leave of the Institute and the people we had met there. We would get our last advice from the doctors and pack all our belongings. We would go back to our day-to-day living. Maybe people would recognize the major changes that Dad had undergone. Maybe they wouldn't. Like getting off of a roller coaster ride at the amusement park, there was both a little disappointment and a little relief that the event was over.

We decided to go to a local Jazz Festival. The Armed Forces Jazz Band was kicking off the day, followed by a list of other great sounding groups. I borrowed two plastic chairs from Bud and Monica at the motel, and put them in the trunk. I packed up our water bottles and sun hats and suntan lotion and we headed to Coachman Park. This was one of those times that I was grateful for handicapped parking. We pulled right down to the water's edge, about a hundred feet from the back of the stage, and parked in the last available handicapped parking space.

I carried our chairs on top of my head as I tried to find the shortest way to the side of the bandstand so Dad didn't have to walk too far. It was hot. Someone called out, "Nice hat!" making fun of my chairs. Finally, we spotted a sliver of shade that I thought would grow as the sun moved to the west, and plopped the chairs down. We were on the very edge of the bandstand, but could see the stage quite clearly. The music had not yet started. Dad limped off towards the nearest Porta-potty. Life seemed normal again. We were doing something that was not associated with the Institute or Dad's therapy.

When Dad came back he was visibly tired. It was so hot. "They didn't have to put that hill between me and the toilets," he complained, as he sat down in the shade. I handed him his water bottle. The hill was a four-foot incline.

"Cool down, Dad. Drink some water." I suggested that we buy some festival T-shirts to take home as gifts. A couple sat down in front of us on low chairs. It seemed odd that we struck up a conversation with these strangers, but we did, as naturally as if they were our next-door neighbors whom we had known for years.

"Where are you from?" the man asked.

"Chicago, but we are staying down here for three weeks so that Dad can go to a clinic that helps stroke victims."

"You mean with physical therapy?" the woman asked.

"No, this doctor is using medications to get remarkable recovery in stroke victims, even those who had strokes many years ago."

The man turned to me, interested. "Most patients don't have any more recovery."

I began to tell him the whole long story about Dad and his fellow patients at the Institute.

"Do you have a phone number?" he asked. "I run a country club over on the Atlantic Coast. We have doctors come in to lecture once a month. Do you think that someone would be willing to talk? We have lots of stroke patients."

"I'm sure someone would," I said. "Are you a computer person? I can give you a web site where you can read about Dr. Hammesfahr's therapy."

"Yes, that would be great."

"It's HNI-Online.com."

We had become the disseminators of information for the Institute. Now, we were the angels passing out the miracles.

But this angel stuff turned out to be harder than we thought. A few weeks later, after Dad had returned to Rock Island, there was an art fair down on Whitehead Street in Key West, and Steve and I wandered the space allotted to the booths. Some were selling dog bonnets, to keep the sun off of a puppy's eyes, while others had items made with incredible craftsmanship, like the tightly woven baskets with horn handles. Rocks wrapped in wire competed with slick gold and tanzanite rings and popcorn stands. The street was full of people. As we walked into a booth with Key West photography, I saw an old woman in a wheel chair, being pushed by her husband through the crowd.

"This is a good opportunity to try the shopping mall hand-off," I told Steve.

"I'll stand over here and watch," he said.

I approached the couple. "Hello," I began. "Did you have a stroke?" I asked the woman.

"Yes, a mild one," she answered, smiling.

"I know a doctor who can help you walk again," I said. "Here's his card." I handed it to her husband, who read it and gave it to her.

"Where is he located?" she asked.

"In Clearwater, Florida."

"Oh honey, you might just as well take this card back. You're wasting it on me. I'm not going all the way to Clearwater for a doctor."

I took my card back. People came from Australia and Europe for this therapy, I thought, but I remained silent and returned to Steve. "It was too far to travel," I said.

"You certainly weren't her angel. Maybe she likes being pushed around by her husband."

"I think she'll come to regret what she just did, and be sorry she didn't take the card."

28
Crossing Bridges
Sunday, October 22
Day Twenty, Medication Day Seventeen

Dad's blood pressure was good in the morning, 142/81. He finished the bottle of milk on his cereal. We drank our allotted six ounces of coffee. I rushed to do one more load of laundry. I had depleted our car ashtray's quarter supply, but I scrounged up two dollars' worth between Dad's pockets and my purse, enough for the washer and dryer.

"Let's take a walk across the bridge," Dad suggested.

"Remember how tired it made you last time? You're not supposed to overdo the exercise. You really complained to Sharon last time."

"It's cool this morning and I think I can make it over to the bench." He was urging me on, instead of my urging him. That was something new.

The tide was high so there weren't many birds, only some Asian fishermen after bait. They stood high on the bridge and flung their circular nets, trapping a few fish with each toss.

A woman was walking towards us. She stopped and leaned on her tall stick to chat. It had been cleaned of all the extraneous bark and had a natural indentation where her hand held it. At five feet, it was taller than her white hair by a good six inches.

"I have to get down to church," she said hoarsely. "They got some food for me. I think it's about two more miles."

"How far have you come already?" I asked. She looked as though she might not make it across the bridge, but the grit in her old eyes told me she would get all the way to wherever she wanted to go.

"A long way. I live in a home now, but I used to live outside, in the woods. I sure miss it." Her skin was so dark and weathered it did not look as though she had been in a home for very long.

"I got laid up with my leg, but it's getting better now." She bent over and pointed to her battle scared shins. "They're working pretty good now." She hoisted herself upright and took off across the bridge.

"If she can do it," Dad said, "so can I." We continued on our way. It was a long walk, but this time Dad was singing.

"Cross over the bridge,
Cross over the bridge,
Leave your evil ways behind you
And true romance will find you.
Brother, cross over the bridge."

Later, Lia called again to confirm our travel plans for Tuesday. Dad bragged about the long walk he'd taken. He didn't complain once about his daughter forcing him to walk miles and miles.

Dad's evening blood pressure was 148/78. He felt great! He walked much better, with a regular gait, and he went much faster. He reached across his body with his bad arm and brushed a bug off of his shoulder. His hand was looser. He could smell himself. When he took a shower he dried his own back using both his right and left hands to pull a towel across it. Before we left the motel, he walked across the bedroom floor in his bare feet without his cane. His balance was much surer. Many things seemed to be coming together and working better.

29
Misgivings and Manicures
Monday, October 23
Day Twenty-one, Medication Day Eighteen

By Dad's appointment that Monday, I had a list of seventeen questions to ask and good news to report.

One of the questions was about an article I'd clipped from the St. Petersburg paper, in which the FDA condemned some popular decongestant medicines. I handed it to Sharon as she was checking Dad's blood pressure.

"Hey, Trouble," she said to Dad, "What's with this blood pressure?" It was 103/60. Too low.

She looked at the headline on the clipping. "Duh," she said, as she handed the clipping to Dr. Raines, who was whizzing by. He got all excited.

"Can I make a copy of this?" he asked. "This is just what we have been saying."

"Keep it," I said.

Dr. Uzo showed up to check the charts.

"How are you feeling?" she asked Dad.

"I felt dizzy this morning," he began.

"You didn't tell me that!" I interrupted. I expected to know every detail of his life, now.

"But I did feel dizzy," he said.

"If it continues, be sure to mention it to your doctor at home," Dr. Uzo advised him. "We may have to change the medications."

"I take this drug, Baclofen. That's what makes me dizzy," Dad said.

Now I saw where he was heading. He hated that drug.

"Why do you take it?" the doctor asked.

"If I don't take it my arm floats all around up in the air. I can't control it and keep it down by my side."

"Stop taking it and see what happens," she advised.

"I am letting go more and I think I have better balance," he admitted. "I sure hate that drug. It will be a pleasure to stop taking it."

"Watch carefully. If your arm no longer floats up in the air, you don't ever need to use it again. Any other changes?"

"I can drink out of a bottle, and feel the right side of my face. And my arm and leg hurt less."

"Good. I want you to change your medication." She handed him a new form with Accupril 0–½–½–1½ written on it. It also said to drink eight ounces of water with an eighth of a teaspoon of salt, 1–0–1–0. I made a mental note to reload the medication box again.

We were at the end of his therapy. How could they still be futzing with his medications at this late date? I thought it was all supposed to be set up and ready to go by the end of three weeks. The next day would be his last day here. What if his medications needed changing immediately when he got home? It would be too complicated for me to explain to my sister and the doctor. I felt my own blood pressure rise along with my panic. My chest constricted.

"Here is a copy of the letter we faxed to your doctor," Dr. Uzo said. "Here are your prescriptions." She handed him paper after paper. "If you are running low on anything I suggest you get it filled here, as it may take a while for your pharmacy back home to get it. They will certainly have to order the magnesium gluconate so be sure to load up on that."

"How do we get the information on the shots and needles for the magnesium?" I asked.

"Here are the two prescriptions, for IV magnesium and for the shot version. A copy of the directions has been sent to your doctor." She thrust another set of papers at dad.

"Do you have the Symptom Chart? It's in the back of the Blue Book. Be sure to fill it out once a week." She continued without waiting for an answer. "Do you have his medication sheet? Be sure to write down any medication changes."

Her instructions went by so fast that she must have sensed my misgivings. "Don't worry. If you have any questions at all, just call us. We are always here on the phones in the afternoons after two o'clock. Just call."

I felt a little better as we left the office.

Rebecca, the special education teacher from New Jersey was just coming out of the magnesium room. "Look what just happened to my hand." She held it aloft joyously. "My fingers have relaxed! I can get a manicure!" I laughed both at her joy and at the frivolous thing she wanted to do. These small things were not small at all when you couldn't do them.

"I want to be able to put on my own bra," Rebecca said. "I know my husband can do it, but I don't want him to. I want to do it."

I could see her point. There was no mystery or magic when a man had to hitch up your bra. You felt more like a horse than a woman.

Dad and I left for our checkout at the physical therapist's office. Dad's humor had soured.

"I haven't progressed very far, have I?" he said. His voice was crabby and negative.

"Why do you say that? I have notes on every improvement."

"I just want to be better. A lot better. A lot faster."

"I know. But it takes time. Your brain is probably fixing something right this minute, you just don't know it yet." I said it to encourage him, but the Institute said it was true.

Cute Alex, the physical therapist, was waiting in the office.

"Any changes?" he asked Dad.

"I can walk better, my arm doesn't hurt as much, and my leg quit hurting, but it tickles." I could see why the doctors asked us to write down the changes. Dad's perceptions of his recovery yo-yoed by the hour.

"Tickles are good," Alex said. "The brain is projecting a different sensation. There is not so much thalamic pain." He started to repeat the tests Dad took on his first visit. "Can you feel this? Look away and point to where I am touching."

Dad pointed to a spot on his hand.

"That's good. You couldn't feel anything before. Now you feel your palm and the side of your hand. Make your hand like mine," he directed, as he made a fist with his right hand.

Dad squeezed his fingers into a semblance of a fist.

"Last time you did the opposite with your fingers. You spread them out. This time is much better. Raise your arm above you head and across to the other side and as far back as you can go."

Alex demonstrated and Dad followed along. "You have more control in your arm than last time, too."

Dad's humor began to improve with all that praise. Emily came in to do the balance tests. He sang,

"I've got high hopes,
I've got high hopes,
I've got high apple pie in the sky hopes.

So if you're feeling blue,
Don't know what to do,
Just remember that ant,
Whoops! There goes another rubber tree plant."

"I love to sing," Emily confessed. "It's my best stress release. I grab a tape of a song that I know and I just belt it out. I don't think of anything else. I concentrate on the words and how I breathe."

"Sing for us," Dad urged.

"I sing only in the car, with the windows rolled up." Dad was busy standing up and sitting down on her hand commands. "Now turn around as fast as you can."

He took little close together steps.

"You'll be dancing soon," I said.

"Step on and off this platform," Emily continued, intent on her work. "Your stance is much narrower than it was before. That means that your balance is better."

Dad walked back and forth across the room with the video camera on to record his progress for posterity. "Balance on your left leg," Emily said. "Eight seconds, twice as long as before. Now try your right leg. Three seconds, that's one second longer than three weeks ago."

"I feel like a performing dog," Dad said.

"I think you did much better," I said, praising him as we headed toward the car when the session was over. "You were much more self-assured and confident in all of the tasks. It looked a lot better to me. Bravo!"

When we got back to the motel, I rearranged the letters on the refrigerator to say DO EXRCIS. For lunch we ate the last of the peanut butter and bananas in sandwiches.

On Monday afternoon, I left Dad at the motel watching CNBC and went to the Institute alone. I had a one o'clock appointment with Dr. Hammesfahr. Aides kept walking by and reassuring me that he was supposed to be there, but they don't know where he was.

There were about twenty new people in the waiting room beginning their three-week sessions. Sharon was listening to a patient who was speaking garbled language, very expressively, but totally without meaning. She grasped his hand and reassured him.

A stocky Hispanic woman was standing next to her husband's wheelchair, talking to another Hispanic woman. "I took only one week off work, not three weeks. Now I have to call and tell her it's going to be three weeks. I may not have a job when I get home."

"There were no other options," said a woman with a thick French accent. "The doctor said, 'I can not tell you it is going to work. I do not see it in other places. But it is not going to hurt.' I asked him what he would do if it were his wife. He replied, 'Probably what you're doing.' So here we are."

Everyone in the room was talking to each other.

"My dad had this stroke three years ago," a good-looking young man confided to me. "Over time you could see the discouragement." He indicated an incredibly sad gray man in a chair. "Last year, he would try to walk. Then he said, 'Why should I do it if I am not going to get any better anyway?' He lost all hope. He was so depressed that I had to I make him come here. I forced him to come. Now he has a willingness to try. Thursday he even tried to exercise a little."

I leaned over to take the man's hands and softly said to him, "You will get better. Everyone gets better." He smiled faintly, but a doubtful look filled his sad eyes.

There was an elegant looking seventy-year-old woman in lavender. Her white hair was coifed and her nails were manicured. Large rings were on her hands and a sour look was on her face. Her arm lay strapped to a board set across the arms of her wheelchair. Her husband wheeled her to the bathroom. They were gone a long time.

The room was a microcosm of stroke injury woes, frozen limbs, depression, hostility, despair, and the tight smiles of those in pain. Many in the room had the worried look of caregivers who wondered if they had done the right thing by coming to the Institute. Their questions echoed silently from chair to chair. Will it work for me? Can I bear getting my hopes up, only to have them crushed with another treatment that does not work? I am not that strong. Maybe I am wasting my money. Maybe I will look like a fool to my friends, to my doctor. What if it works, what if…it works and my spouse can speak again or walk again or laugh again. What if they are angry or depressed when they do speak?

Sharon called me into the room. "Here is one of the caregivers for a patient who is leaving today. Robin, would you talk to these new people?" She pointed to me in the anteroom and I agreed.

I was in my milieu. I had not taught classrooms full of students for thirty years for naught. I knew how to give an extemporaneous speech. This was an opportunity to get my message across and I wouldn't miss it. I began.

"I have been here for three weeks with my father. I know how you feel right now. I know you are afraid to hope, for fear that the fall will be too far if you fail. What lies ahead is unknown. Each of you will struggle with individual problems. But you can relax a little bit. Everyone I've seen who follows this treatment gets better. In the three weeks I have been here, I have seen people who could not talk begin to speak. I have seen people who always carried their arms clenched against their chests with that tight pained look relax their arms and smile again. Some people walk again. Some get their personalities and energy back first.

"My father got his memory and his sense of humor back first. Now he can make jokes and remember the names of his friends. He doesn't forget ideas in mid-conversation. His arm is relaxing and he can walk better. He has much less pain. He used to cry himself to sleep at night because the pain was so intense. This week he stopped taking Ibuprofen because his pain was almost gone. We go home tomorrow, but that does not mean that this treatment is over. Dad will continue to get better and better as long as he stays on the treatment. So will you.

"You all had the courage to take this chance. Someone, or some idea, or some magical sign, got you here. You are brave. You are people who take risks and you will succeed. Stay the course. Don't give up. What you think are miracles happen here, every day, the result of common medications. The real miracle is that you had the courage to come. The real miracle is that you still have the hope that you can get better. Drink your water!" I waved good-by.

I felt as though I'd been back in the classroom giving my students inspirational messages about why the homework assignment I'd just given them was the most important writing assignment of their short lives. It felt good. I felt useful again in the old way, pontificating on a subject about which I was sure.

One of my former students, Esme Codell, the author of *Educating Esme*, had recently sent me an e-mail about a book she was writing, *Sahara Special*, that gave me the same feeling. It seemed that I was going in circles with this book, she wrote. "I had so much material, but it looked like my son's bedroom, a pretty mess. I stayed up late and finally composed an outline that I liked. You were with me in spirit. You made us write all those 'Ms. Robinson's Handy-Dandy-Five-Paragraph-Outline' formats from the short stories we read. I thought, why is she making us write one every day? Fifteen years later, I know why, and I am so thankful. I don't know how anybody can write a page without a Ms. Robinson somewhere in her past."

My father taught me the five-paragraph outline form when I was fourteen years old. We had moved to a new town again and I didn't know anyone. In the doldrums of late summer, he pointed out a newspaper essay contest to me. It was the first essay I ever wrote and it was all over the place. Dad sat me down and showed me how to organize my meandering prose. Paragraph One - main idea with three supporting ideas, briefly stated, Paragraph Two – first supporting idea with proof, Paragraph Three – second supporting idea with proof, Paragraph Four – third supporting idea with proof, Paragraph Five, restate main idea and three supporting ideas. His concept was that every piece of writing was organized in much the same way. I owed him beyond all comprehension, as I used that format teaching every student I had from Educationally Mentally Handicapped to Advanced Placement for thirty years.

Dr. Raines took me into his office for a little goodbye chat and to try to answer any questions I had for Dr. Hammesfahr. I grilled him.

"Are there other areas besides stroke that have been explored in relationship to this treatment?"

"Yes," he said. Dr. Hammesfahr started out working with closed head injuries, migraine headache patients, cerebral palsy patients, women with silicone breast implants, and ADHD and ADD kids. All were neurological diseases that related to vascular constriction, Parkinson's, MS, seizures, epilepsy, dyslexia, Tourette's, autism, brain injuries, spinal cord injuries, and coma seem to respond to this treatment. They all seemed to have many of the same symptoms, so Dr. Hammesfahr concluded that they must have something in common. He started doing TCDs (Transcranial Dopplers or ultrasounds) on every patient. He found that the common denominator was the constricted blood vessels. Eliminating their spasms was the beginning."

"Are there any other areas where this treatment is effective?" I asked.

"Donna has had improvement as a post polio patient, but she is the only one who has tried it. It also seems to help the hardening of the arteries of diabetics."

"You once told me that a few people do not get better," I said. "Who are they and why do they not get better?"

"Some are not compliant. They don't follow the directions or take their medicines. They are very negative about their life and their disease, and they quit taking medications because they are so depressed. Some don't see changes, even though changes take place. One woman claimed that she had not changed because she had not got the use of her arm back. But she had not been able to walk more than twelve steps before, and now she could walk two miles. People are all different. For a very few, the stroke is so large that nothing happens. Everything is dead already. With our current patients, almost a hundred percent get better.

"What is going to happen in the future? Shouldn't everyone know about this?"

"We will continue here at the Institute. We would like to teach every doctor in the world to do this. But that takes money. We are going to try to start a not-for-profit organization. One problem is that Dr. Hammesfahr is not affiliated with any university. He may never get into some professional journals because he won't do double blind studies."

"What are those?"

"Studies where some patients are given placebos and others are given an identical dose of medications. When everyone he treats gets better, how would he decide who gets the treatment and who does not? He knows that every patient who gets treatment will get better and everyone who does not get it will have no change. How can he deny treatments for a statistical study? He won't do it. It's not ethical. We have a hundred years of data that shows stroke patients don't get better after the first few months. This treatment gets them better and the longer they stay on the treatment the more improvement they get. He is not part of the mainstream research world. It is simply wrong to give a placebo in this situation.

"Also, with this kind of treatment giving all of the patients the same dose of medication would be dangerous. The right dose varies from patient to patient and even varies within that patient over time. It has to be customized for each individual.

"But he is listed on the Nobel Prize web site. He is the only individual doctor on the page; everyone else is associated with a university or major institution. He is an individual doctor who has discovered something new. It is not an easy position."

"It seems so logical."

Dr. Raines sighed, as if to say you know how the world is. "There is another thing we think is happening. We now have patients who are coming back after more than three years on the medications. They are having significant repair to their blood vessels. Evidently the fibroblasts, the scar tissues that form inside the blood vessels, are disappearing. This is an excellent situation as more and more recovery is occurring, even after two or three years. It means that there is a change in the lining of the vessels. We don't know how much is due to remodeling of the vessels and how much is due to vascular opening. Diabetics especially, who have fifty percent more hardening of the arteries than the average person, could benefit from this treatment if it is repairing the blood vessels."

Dr. Raines talked a mile a minute about his computer program that was a spreadsheet of patient recovery. I got out of there an hour later and headed to the motel to pack up for the next day's return to Chicago.

I was exhausted again and worried about leaving the Institute and handling Dad's illness without the support it provided. Dad asked for his pills and I started to cry. "Don't ask me for anything more," I barked. "You are capable of getting them yourself." I slammed out the door into the cool evening air.

The sun was setting, but it had moved south and was hardly visible from the fishing pier, so I walked out along the sidewalk and across the bridge at Stevenson Creek. The path along the bay was busy with dog walkers and bike riders. Cars pulled into the parking lot and couples sat inside, kissing and watching the sun sink while escaping the cool weather. I walked down the path as the skies turned the water lavender and pink. There were no clouds when I stopped to watch the small white herons gorge on minnows along the shoreline. I tried a huge Cosmic Sigh, putting more oxygen in my system, people at the Institute would say. I stood up straight and tried to concentrate on my breathing instead of feeling sorry for myself about how much I had to do each day, and guilty because Dad's blood pressure was still not stabilized and the doctors were still changing his medications.

A bird's trill interrupted my silence, insistent and repetitive. I looked for the bird in the small tree before me. "Trrruuuupp, trruuuuupp, squa, squa, squa," it sang. I spotted it on a top branch. It was plump and beige and not at all afraid. I crept closer and closer until I was within three feet away of it. It looked right at me and continued to blare its song. I searched for another bird and listened for answering chirp thinking that a sweetheart serenade was about to ensue.

A woman stopped behind me and pulled up her binoculars. "It's a shrike, I think," she said. "It's talking to you." She lowered the binoculars and walked on.

That settled into my brain a few seconds before I realized what it meant. The bird talking to me was my mother in another one of her crazy bird disguises. This was getting really bizarre, but I listened. I cleared my mind to receive whatever this messenger from Mom wanted to tell me. I listened to the melody to see if there were any words that popped into my head. Nothing. The bird kept staring straight at me with its "rat-a-tat-tat squa, squa, squa" song. "Relax," I told myself out loud. "Make your mind empty." That was it. Relax. Mother was telling me to let go of my anger and guilt and enjoy the beauty of nature around me. I needed to be patient with Dad's medications and give them time to work. This was the right path. Trust the doctors. Relax. The tension drained from my face and neck and I felt better.

"I got it," I said. The bird kept on singing. "I got it, Mom. Thank you." There was a pause in the bird's song, then it flitted down to a lower branch and I could no longer see it. It stopped singing. I walked home as the orange sun sank through the cloudless sky into the bay.

Sometimes I thought that listening for advice from the aviary population of the world was truly dumb. Surely anyone who heard me talking to the birds would assume I was coo-coo. But in another way, stopping to listen to the birds wasn't such a bad idea after all. It offered a little silence for inside the head and created a space between problems and their solutions. It was a way to balance emotions with duties. Mother always liked birds. She named me Robin. Why wouldn't she try to talk to me through my namesakes? I liked the idea. Maybe there were guardian angels and she was mine. It had symmetry, even if it was silly.

Dad was waiting in front of the TV set. "I'm sorry for storming out," I said as I kissed him on the cheek.

"That's okay, honey," he said evenly. "I got the meds myself."

I began packing his clothes. The closet was stuffed with all the new shorts and pants he'd acquired in Clearwater. I used this speedy system: I put all the clothes on hangers on the bed, removed the hangers and then folded the clothes into a giant roll, and put it in the suitcase. Everything else went around the edges. I got finished fast.

We decided to return to the lovely restaurant where we'd had dinner the first night we'd arrived in Clearwater, 'bon appetit.'

"You ready?" I asked. "Are we going to celebrate tonight! I think this has been a very successful three weeks." "I'm ready when you are," he said. Then he sang,

"When the red, red robin goes bob, bob, bobbin along,

They'll be no more sobbin', when she comes bobbin along.

Wake up, wake up, you sleepyheads,

Get up, get up, get out of bed.

Cheer up, cheer up,

The night has fled,

Live, love, laugh and be happy."

Just as I was finished and ready to leave for dinner, the phone rang. It was Steve. "I have a bit of bad news," he said.

I hate it when people start out like that. I realized that Steve was trying to cushion the news, but so far, my expectations of bad news had been far worse than anything anyone had ever told me. My greatest fear has always been that my children would die before I did, so that was my first thought.

"Who died?"

"No one. It's not that bad."

"What is it?"

"I got my prostate biopsy from the doctor today. I have cancer."

"Oh, no." I couldn't think beyond it. "This *is* bad," I said. "This is not good."

"I made an appointment to see the doctor on Wednesday when you get home. He wants to discuss treatment and I want you to be there with me."

My dad heard the anguish in my voice and came into the room.

"I am so sorry. I am so sorry. Oh no," I said dumbly. Dad looked worried so I put my hand over the phone and whispered, "Steve has prostate cancer." Dad knew what that was about. He had it, too. I had been through all the options with him when he was first diagnosed.

There was no easy cure for prostate cancer. The three choices were: take the prostate out surgically and risk incontinence or impotence, or both, and some patients died on the operating table; radiate it and risk impotence or damage to other nearby organs with the added worry of reoccurrence of the cancer; or try hormones and watch the genitals shrink to nothing, knowing the cancer was still lurking there. There was no cure, only postponement.

Doctors tried to be up beat and stress the positive to keep patients from depression. They explained, but obfuscated the negative. With cancer, everyone pretended. The good cheer was hollow. The unsaid was behind what the doctors said. "It's not as bad as you think. Lots of people survive a long time with this type of cancer. You should do quite well." But there was no miracle man waiting in the wings with a new medication for prostate cancer.

Strokes could be fixed. Cancer lurked, waiting for its next opportunity. Cancer doctors' waiting rooms were not filled with joy and laughter like Dr. Hammesfahr's were. At the Institute office everyone really was getting better, no one got worse. With cancer, everyone got worse sooner or later.

Our celebration soured. We smiled, but they were worried, nervous smiles. We watched the sun set, all gold and pink, and contemplated the brevity and the beauty of life. I thought about how deeply sad my father was that my mother was gone and how disturbed he was that he couldn't have been whole for her, if she were alive. He'd learned to live with it. We would, as well.

30
Medicine, Not Miracles
Tuesday, October 24
Day Twenty-two, Medication Day Nineteen

We were due at the doctor's office by nine o'clock for Dad's last ultrasound, final blood pressure check, and for one last visit with the doctor du jour. In the morning, Dad was tired and sore. He got up at five-thirty and said he couldn't sleep anymore. When we got to the Institute for our appointment, Dad was slow. His arms jerked more. He missed two steps on the front porch and had to mount them one by one. He said he was cold. He had refused to drink any water because of the flight scheduled in the afternoon.

Behind us an old man came in carrying his wife's big white purse. She struggled up the steps behind him. I had never seen them before. Sharon whizzed by. "Your purse matches your shoes," she said to him. There was a slight pause and then the room erupted into laugher as the man realized what she actually said. He looked down at his white tennis shoes and smiled as he held the door for his wife. Sharon and Summer Rose Wright raced back and forth.

Sharon put us in an office to take Dad's blood pressure. I was surprised that it was so high considering how he felt. It was 119/66.

"If a snake were here I could walk under his belly," Dad told her.

"If you keep that negative attitude going you will have to crawl under the snake's belly," she teased him.

"You won't let me do anything. I can't even cross my legs," he teased right back.

"That's right!" She gave him a small glass of water with some salt in it. "Drink this."

"Will it make me larger or smaller?"

"You're not Alice," I said.

Dr. Raines sped by. "There goes the Great Father!" Sharon quipped. "You get an ultrasound today," she told Dad. "Debbie is waiting for you."

Debbie sat Dad in the wing chair and pulled his blood vessel pictures from the machine.

"They don't look too much different from last time," I said.

"Sometimes it takes a few months for them to look better. They are a little lower than before. That's good." She tucked them in his file.

Sharon took his blood pressure again. It was 119/76. "That's a little better. The salt is working."

Dr. Uzo stopped to check the chart and talk to Dad. "How are you feeling? Any changes?" she asked.

"I feel tired this morning."

This was the last time that we would talk to a doctor. I was terrified of being alone with responsibility for Dad's care, especially since I was not going to be in Rock Island with him. I couldn't control what was going to happen. It might get messed up. I decided to make some comforting lists while Dr. Uzo was reviewing the charts. I started with a list of the lists that I was going to make.

1. Made Dad a schedule of medications
2. Make a list of things for my sister
3. Make a list for the Fort Armstrong Hotel
4. Make a list for Dad

5. Make a list for Dad's doctor in Rock Island
6. Load all of his pills for the next week
I felt better, already.

"If you are worried, just ask him the four questions," Dr. Uzo said. "Who is the president? What day of the week is it? What month is it? What year is it? And what did you have to eat last night?"

"That's five." I said.

"Leave out, the president," she suggested. "You can call us any afternoon, for anything. We will be here to answer your questions."

Sharon stuck her head around the corner. "Dr. Hammesfahr is here to talk to you today. When you finish with Dr. Uzo, go into his office and wait. He'll be right downstairs."

I looked at my watch. It was now eleven and we had to check out of the motel and be at the airport by one. Too much was happening too fast. I hated to rush. We moved to the other office. Dad came in with me.

Dr. Hammesfahr appeared in the open necked blue shirt that matched his eyes. He still looked a bit like a college professor, rumpled and hurriedly dressed as though dressing was not an important part of his day.

"Sorry about yesterday. I got held up looking at a larger facility that would give us more space."

The Institute was often full of people so I understood why he was looking for more space. Steve says that I always want to know far more than I need to know. Now my school teacher 'I have to know everything," voice took over.

"You're young. You must have started studying neurology when you were a babe. How did you learn so much?

"I have been interested in neurology since I was a kid. My parents tried to dissuade me by saying that this was too difficult a career with long hours and frequent emotional trauma. To discourage me they advised me to do volunteer work for Matheny Hospital and School for the severely disabled, thinking that I would see first-hand how emotionally demanding medicine was.

"My scout master thought it would be a good idea to establish a scout troop at the hospital in order to satisfy our Eagle Scout requirements for a community service project. The children at the school all had major physical and developmental disabilities. The Scout troop could give these institutionalized kids a sense of self-worth and independence as we worked on craft projects with them in the same way that it did it for boys all over the world. The patients all got Boy Scout shirts and hats, and the school personnel dressed them before our weekly meetings.

"The first time our troop walked into the room with the kids I was overwhelmed by the sights and smells. These kids were in bad shape. They looked weird and angular. Their bodies and muscles were contorted or contracted. When they saw the rest of my Scout troop they got excited and began making grunting sounds and flailing their arms about. They were obviously very needy.

"I was shocked. I left the room and threw up. After, as I went around the room talking to the kids, I began to focus on their needs and I saw them in an entirely different way as individuals. They needed to be noticed. They needed someone to pay attention to them. They desperately needed to communicate. Some of them were able to spell out words by moving letters around on boards, but it was a huge effort to get even a single word out.

"They were proud to wear the Scout shirts and hats. They enjoyed the flag ceremony that began each meeting. They looked forward to our weekly meetings and I looked forward to seeing them each week.

"I worked with these kids at this red brick hospital in New Jersey once a week over the next year. The experience had the opposite effect than the one my parents anticipated. I grew attached to these damaged kids. These children faced the world with incredible hope. Despite their terrible infirmities, they continued to try. And they did it with good spirits. They were good kids trapped in terrible bodies. It confirmed for me that I wanted to help these children. It was emotionally difficult to work with them, but they were the reason I chose medicine."

I checked out my Dad. He was quiet but interested. "My youngest son completed his school service requirement by volunteering for a week at Miscordia a school for disabled children in Chicago, and he returned home shaken by the experience."

"Your parents would have approved of *his* reaction," Dad smiled.

"You went to Northwestern University in Chicago, didn't you?" I asked glancing at the diplomas on the wall.

"Yeah, I had a great schooling experience there. I was admitted in a special program which accepted me directly into medical school from high school. I graduated from their Honors Program in Medical Education in 1982. At the time, Northwestern University Medical School was ranked first in the nation in clinical medicine and in the top ten overall. I went on to do my residency at The Medical College of Virginia in neurosurgery. It was one of two "Centers for Excellence" for the treatment of brain and head injury. I was a practicing neurosurgeon in training there.

"How did you deduce that vasodilators would make stroke patients recover?" I asked.

"I noticed when I was working in surgery that each doctor had his own set of protocols for patients. Patients with identical diagnosis got different treatment, depending on the doctor and what treatment had worked for him in the past. I thought if we could use some of the new technology available in the hospital to measure the patient's vital signs during surgery, treatment would be more objective."

I was intrigued. "So you invented a new technique?"

"I used the new machines in a different way. A surgeon in the operating room could see what was working immediately and make changes if they were not working. I wanted to apply this new skill so doctors could have more information during surgery and during treatment thereby improving patient recovery. Florida had a serious malpractice problem. This system would give patients better care *and* help protect doctors from malpractice suits."

"You're not a neurosurgeon now. What happened?"

"In retrospect, I never would have been involved in this amazing new therapy if fate had not changed the direction of my work. I was given one of those optimistic 'opportunities for growth' in the form of a major setback.

"The first year I worked in surgery, my hands became red and inflamed from wearing latex gloves. I ignored the condition. By the third year they were covered with red and scaling skin. During the fourth year we began to pour oil into gloves and let my hands soak for a while until they could move normally. The hospital tried to help me with this allergy by ordering latex-free gloves from Switzerland, but by that time I had become sensitized to soaps and other chemicals. My hands festered and crusty scabs formed over the sore places. It wasn't long before I could not bend my fingers. Minuscule work on a patient's brain was out of the question. My career in neurosurgery was shattered.

"I asked the Medical College of Virginia if I might switch to neurology and, although they did not usually allow it, they agreed. I tried to convince myself that this change would be good. My sister-in-law had multiple sclerosis. That gave me an added incentive to study neurology.

"The more I worked in neurology the more interesting it became. I ended up with extensive experience in two medical fields, neurology and neurosurgery. I was particularly interested in the work in the Intensive Care Unit where they were monitoring blood flow equilibrium and blood flow within the brain. Again, life seemed on track.

"The time I'd spent in the operating room taught me how to use sophisticated machinery to measure changes in blood flow in a patient's brain. As it turned out, it was a very important skill in the treatment of neurological diseases."

"Is that what you are doing when you test Dad with the ultrasound machine?"

"Yes. After I finished residency, my wife and I moved to Florida. I was a licensed physician, Board Certified in Neurology and Pain Management. I began working at St. Petersburg Medical Clinic, training groups of technicians and doctors to use the advanced technological techniques that I had pioneered in order to regulate their patient's recovery. It turned out that these machines, which are sensitive to diagnosing when things are going wrong in the nervous system, are also good for identifying when things are going right in the nervous system. I decided to use them to look for when things were starting to get better, sort of an early detection system for finding the right treatment.

"Most technical assessment tools are not used for monitoring as I was doing. Despite the fact that this was a new way of using the machines, private insurance companies paid for these sessions as a preventive measure against malpractice suits. Then, because of legislative changes, the crisis in the insurance industry was resolved. Soon after that, the insurance codes changed and insurance companies ceased paying for the training sessions. I was left with a lot of trained technical personnel and expensive machinery."

"So you had to start all over again," I said.

"I set up a private practice in Clearwater. I moved all of the expensive machinery that I had used in my last job and installed it in my office. These technologies were new to the West Coast of Florida and rare in the country as a whole. This advanced level of work resulted in speaking engagements and teaching sessions on a professional level at major universities and regional centers around the country. I was appointed a reviewer for the Department of Education which meant that I reviewed university grant requests for new technology and treatment modalities. Later, I was asked to function as Chief Reviewer. I was certified by the State of Florida for the evaluation of disability.

"That's impressive," I said noticing that Dad was still all ears, but not saying much.

"I used the ultrasound machines and other technology in my private practice. I also began working with the Clearwater Community Hospital testing, and with patients who filed claims against insurance agencies for spinal cord injuries resulting from automobile accidents. We could tell whether there had been an injury or not by doing tests with the new technology I had been using. I looked at more than a thousand serious cases a year. Then the automobile manufacturers installed air bags. Within four years, injuries dropped from a thousand cases a year to thirty cases a year. Air bags work really well.

"At that time, I was treating a group of patients in my private practice who were completely disabled and severely brain damaged from a variety of wounds and accidents. They were all on Social Security Disability and had been on it for from five to twenty years. They had constant debilitating migraines that they had been told by other doctors were untreatable. Their pain was terrible to see. More good people in terrible bodies.

"I had a lot of sophisticated equipment in my office. Since it is rare to have all that technology in one place, when some new medications for migraine came on the market I brought a number of these brain injured patients into the office and tried a tiny dose of each new medicine while monitoring them using the sophisticated machinery, to test the results. I thought while no one drug would alleviate the migraines, I could create a cocktail of drugs that might help the patients with their terrible and debilitating pain.

"I examined each patient with these tests: a computerized Electroencephalogram (EEG), a Brainstem

Auditory Evoked Potentials test, a Somatosensory Evoked Potentials test, a Visual Evoked Potentials test, and a Transcranial Doppler. Patients received repetitive clinical neurological examinations, sometimes as often as every three minutes. We'd take a pre-test, administer medications and then do post tests to see the exact effect of the medication on each individual patient.

"The two migraine drugs that I tried were new on the market. I was very cautious, so I started the doses in such small quantities that they couldn't possibly hurt any of the patients. The first one I tried was Imitrex, which is a vascular constrictor used for treating acute migraines. I tried tiny doses while I monitored the patients to see what the medication would do. The patient's blood vessels narrowed and their migraines went away, but they actually worsened neurologically, and their test results showed worsening of the abnormal activity in the brain. When the drug wore off, the migraines returned.

"Next, I tried Toradol, another medicine used for treating migraines. These tests results showed improved and sometimes normal brain activity after we gave the patients the medicine. The patients' migraines also went away, but the drug worked in an entirely different way in the body. It expanded the blood vessels. Their neurological symptoms disappeared and their test results showed normal brain activity.

"If I had started with a protocol "normal" dose I would have failed because the normal doses would have made the blood vessels constrict. My extreme caution produced amazing results.

"I thought we would see one patient respond better to a medication on one set of tests, and another respond better to a different medication measured by a different set of tests. That would imply that those specific medications would each be a little bit effective, but combined they would be very effective. However, I did not expect to see the patients get significantly better right in the middle of these tests. Amazingly, they did."

Dr. Hammesfahr leaned forward over his big wooden desk looking as though he had just seen the results for the first time that moment. His eyes glazed over as he remembered that powerful moment.

"They did it that quickly?" I could see my father wishing that he had been one of those lucky ones. His recovery was remarkable, but less dramatic.

"Patients with severe brain injuries, who hadn't been able to walk unassisted for five or ten years, suddenly got up off our examining tables and took off across the room.

"Right before our eyes, their whole personalities changed. Their memories improved dramatically. Their responses to other people improved. Their headaches went away. Patients who were having almost constant seizures, a brain injury side effect, stopped having seizures. As soon as the medications wore off, the patients regressed. It happened in the space of fifteen minutes or forty-five minutes or an hour, depending on how long the particular medication remained active in their bodies.

"We found that the medications that were not supposed to get rid of pain, because they caused dilation of blood vessels, were the ones that actually did alleviate the pain.

"We learned that conventional migraine therapy was wrong.

"We found that rather than making the blood vessels constrict further, the therapy should be designed to make the blood vessels dilate in order to make the original constriction go away. While constricting the blood vessels temporarily stopped the headache, it perpetuated the migraine cycle. Think of the constriction as a muscle spasm in a blood vessel."

Dr. Hammesfahr pulled out his pen and a pad of paper and began drawing a crude picture of a constricted blood vessel as he spoke.

"A constriction, like a rubber band around a blood vessel, resulted in less blood flow behind the constricted spasm. In order to compensate for the loss of blood that was unable to get through the constricted muscle spasm, the blood vessel expanded beyond the constriction. The constriction *caused* the expansion. If a physician treated the expansion without treating the constriction, the migraine simply re-occurred. When I treated the constriction, the blood vessels beyond the constriction had no reason to expand and -they returned to normal. The migraines did not reoccur.

"This was a revolutionary discovery.

"We also discovered that most brain injury patients were essentially in a state of chronic migraine with insufficient blood flow to the brain. Intermittently, the headache came on as another symptom of the migraine, but the constriction that aggravated the memory loss, caused personality changes, and neurological and balance problems was present, to some degree, all of the time. The fluctuations in these symptoms corresponded to the fluctuations in the blood vessels' diameter. The medications affected a wide variety of patients' symptoms, not just their headaches.

"Over a period of many months, using our sophisticated technology, we tried out every single blood vessel medication we could find. We performed detailed tests until we learned which ones worked, how they worked, and how to anticipate and avoid their dangers. Ultrasounds (Transcranial Dopplers) turned out to be most effective tool for measuring the changes in blood vessels.

"Within three months, ninety percent of the first thirty patients we treated went off Social Security Disability. Many returned to work. They no longer needed any medicine for headaches. They rejoined their joyful families.

"I began to wonder exactly what I had discovered."

"Millions of people have terrible migraines. Their doctors should know this. It would prevent so much pain." I wondered why this method of relieving pain had not been adopted by every doctor in the country immediately.

"I didn't know how to get this information out. My wife and I were scheduled for a vacation to Hawaii and I vowed to stop thinking about this for a little while. We had rented a condo with views of the incredible Hawaiian landscape. Our place was on the top of a high hill with a long slope down to the Pacific Ocean. I relaxed and my mind felt blue like the water.

"I was looking at the ocean through the kitchen window and watching it pick up glints of sunlight when one of those glints lit up my head. I had an inspiration in front of that kitchen sink in Hawaii. It felt amazing. One little cataclysmic idea. It was so powerful that I felt touched by something bigger than myself. I was not an overly religious man before this happened to me, but now, I think that I was blessed that moment. It's as if a miracle occurred that would change my life and the lives of millions. It was a thought and like a great mathematical proof, the thought alone was so simple. I am a neurologist. Neurologists study nerves, but it is *not* the nerves, it's the blood vessels.

"I often wonder, Why me? Why did a practicing physician in a backwater town discover this new therapy? Why not a researcher in a major institution? In a major city? But there it was. I got the breakthrough."

"Doctors and researchers must get so involved in thinking inside the box that they can't imagine any other way," Dad said. "It was like that in my profession."

"By treating the blood vessels, we could help the nerves to recover. It was the blood vessels that control the recovery of the nerves. Unbeknownst to me, I was marching straight towards a revolution in neurology. That miraculous paradigm shift in thinking set me on the journey to this innovative new therapy.

"When I got home, I began serious observation of *all* my patients who exhibited the same symptoms, whether they had a spinal cord injury or ADD and I started serious search for the best medications to open their blood vessels."

"There are so many different diseases involved," I said. "Don't they all have different ways of treating them?"

"We discovered that they are all, in part, a vascular disease, not strictly neurological or cardiac. They are all a part of the same problem and the problem is vascular." He sat back and spread his arms and smiled. Then he leaned forward again.

"Another interesting thing occurred shortly after I treated the patients with severe migraine headaches. I was asked by the Plaintiff Attorneys to examine a number of silicone breast implant patients suffering from neurological problems. These patients needed neurological testing for a Federal Court case. The Federal Judge had issued a set of protocols for the neurological testing. There were only two physicians in the Tampa Bay area who were qualified to do this testing and I was one of them. Hundreds of patients were funneled to the two of us.

"After treating more than twenty-five hundred cases of severe brain injury and other neurological diseases, I discovered that I couldn't tell the difference on the ultrasound between the blood vessels of the patients with brain injury and the blood vessels of the patients with the silicone breast implants. They looked much the same. Their EEG's looked the same as well.

"I realized that I was examining a variety of neurological problems with these women, but not only did their ultrasounds and EEGs look the same, they all had symptoms similar to the patients with brain injuries that I had successfully treated. They were histrionic. They had had personality changes and were hostile and depressed. They were dyslexic. Light and sound hurt them. Their balance was poor and they all had terrible migraine headaches.

"These women were too disabled to work, so, like the migraine headache patients, I could keep them in the Institute for eight hours of treatment. I monitored them with the ultrasound while I adjusted the doses of medications for each patient individually.

"Gradually, by observation, I discovered which medications worked best for most of the women. When I used those medications, their symptoms disappeared and the ultrasounds which measured their blood flow, improved. Some women got rid of their headaches in just a few minutes. "

"Great research project," Dad said.

"I did not think of it as doing research. I was simply observing and treating patients. If it worked, I did it again. If it didn't work, I tried something else. There was a therapeutic window for each patient that was unique. If they got the right dose, they got better. If they got a dose that was too high or too low, the blood vessels narrowed and they did not get better. In doing this, I found out that the correct dose was different for each patient.

"I also found out that a patient's blood vessels had to be re-programmed to stay open. This was a process. It took medication that would remain consistent in the patient's body. It also took time for the blood vessels to heal the scar tissue that had built up in them. If there was neurological damage, it took a longer time for the nerves to re-grow. Woody, it will take time for your blood vessels to heal."

"I'm old. I don't have a whole lot of time," Dad said as he shifted his weight with his cane.

"These women were all seeing psychologists, Dr. Robinson. Soon, I began getting calls from the patients' doctors asking questions. They said their patients' I.Q.'s were going up. Their symptoms were gone. They wanted to know what I was doing.

"The leaching silicone had evidently made their blood vessels constrict. When their blood vessels opened up, the patients lost their symptoms. Interestingly, when the women with silicone breast implants got better, they all got better in the same pattern. We saw their personalities change and they became less hostile and depressed. They lost the pain caused by sound and light. Their balance got better and their headaches went away. Then their language and dyslexia improved."

"How thrilling for you," I said.

"And for them," said Dad ever interested in others.

"The same psychologists in town who were treating these brain injury and breast implant patients also were treating children with learning disabilities. Because some of the symptoms were the same, the psychologists started sending me these learning disabled patients.

"The first two I treated were young adults. They were socially isolated and had no friends. They couldn't follow a joke or understand a punch line. They seemed bright but couldn't remember how to use a cash register. They had many of the same symptoms as the other patients I treated. Not surprisingly, I found the same ultrasound results, severe narrowing of their blood vessels. They improved quickly with treatment, gaining over thirty IQ points within a month.

"Many children were subsequently referred to me. This work was successfully extended to patients with Attention Deficit Hyperactive Disorder, Attention Deficit Disorder, dyslexia, emotional and behavioral disturbances, Tourette's syndrome, and autism. I have treated more than five hundred children to date."

"When did you start to treat stroke patients?" Dad asked.

"The first stroke patient that I ever treated with this new concept was the nurse Robin mentioned reading about in the United Airline ad. Perhaps the reason she was not as hesitant to try the therapy as Robin, was because she was a relative. By this time I had used this therapy on thousands of patients with brain injuries, but none with strokes, although many of the symptoms were the same and I thought it would work.

"My wife's aunt, Mitzi Harrell, was near retirement but still looked like Peter Pan. She had short gray hair, a quick, ready smile and enough optimism to sustain a hospital full of nurses. Because she was a nurse (Associate Dean of Nursing at the Presbyterian School of Nursing in Charlotte, North Carolina), she and I had talked about the work that I was doing with brain injured patients long before she had a stroke and she understood how the therapy worked. When she had a stroke shortly after cardiac surgery she called me at the Institute."

Once Dr. Hammesfahr got started on a story, he rushed through the telling of it as though he was driven to pack as much information into as few minutes as possible. I sat back and listened to him go.

"Mitzi had expected to go on permanent disability from her job but before she did, she decided to come down here to try this new therapy. She was sometimes confused and often unable to converse. To enter the Institute she had to be held up by others. After completing her neurological work-up, I began medications.

"Within fifteen minutes of her first dose of medication, she was able to walk forty feet without any assistance. Then she went outside the Institute and ran across the back yard. She had only minor weakness in her shoulder and her leg. Her speech became normal with only an occasional stutter or word substitution. Her confusion disappeared. In the next fifteen minutes, as the medication wore off, she reverted to her previous state. We spent the next few days getting her dosages correct so that her recovery would last all day. By day three she could step onto a boat from off a dock, without assistance. She went home after four days.

"Instead of going on permanent disability when she returned to North Carolina, she returned to full duties at the School of Nursing. She was promoted to Dean of the School within two months. My wife's family was very happy." "Nothing like impressing the in-laws." Dad laughed, probably thinking of his own efforts with Mom's parents.

"Six months later, a local physician who knew of my work in brain injury referred a house painter named Ron Clark. Twelve strokes had left this thin man with the lopsided smile completely paralyzed on the right side of his body. He had spent a full year in the VA Hospital and three additional years paralyzed, without improvement, before coming to the Institute. He was unable to walk without heavy braces and spent much of his time in a wheelchair. He had poor concentration and memory, but a strong will.

"Six weeks after beginning treatment Ron was moving the right side of his body. In another six weeks his memory and concentration improved. Within six months, he resumed his job as a house painter and was climbing ladders to the tops of three story buildings. He regained fine motor control and began playing his guitar again. He got off Social Security disability, got his contracting license, and opened his own firm in Clearwater. A year later, as a labor of love, he painted our building."

This man could easily be a university professor, I thought. He could fill up an hours lecture without any problem at all.

"The third case Robin mentioned was a neurologist and stroke and brain injury specialist with thirty-three years of experience, Dr. William Scott Russell, Jr. In his practice he had treated thousands of stroke patients. He had first-hand knowledge of the procedures protocol we were using because he had peer reviewed a paper I wrote concerning my treatment protocol using vasodilators. He knew exactly what we were doing at the Institute and was impressed with our work.

PEELING THE ONION   240

"In 1996 Dr. Russell experienced a stroke. When he awoke one morning, he was confused. He went to work and had difficulty speaking and writing. He asked a technician in his office to run an EEG to confirm his self-diagnosis of acute stroke. Because he was impressed with our work at the Institute, he presented himself for treatment on the same day he experienced the stroke.

"I performed a Transcranial Doppler on Dr. Russell and administered nitroglycerin to dilate his blood vessels. Ten minutes after the nitroglycerin was administered, his symptoms disappeared. We adjusted his medications and Dr. Russell felt that he had total recovery from the stroke. He has not had a return of the deficits.

We were able to get increased collateral blood flow to the area of a stroke called a penumbra. This larger area of brain tissue around the center of the stroke was not receiving enough blood flow for the nerves to work properly. We used standard anti-hypertensive blood pressure medicines to do this. The medications increased the size of the blood vessels in the area of the stroke, thus increasing blood flow to areas damaged by the stroke. We individualized the medications to each patient. Mitzi's medications were different from Ron's and Ron's different from Dr. Russell's.

"Those cases did impress me," I said, sneaking a glance at my watch and worrying about our closely approaching flight.

"After that I began treating a large number of stroke patients and I decided to document the recovery of a group of them. Over the course of more than a year I watched and recorded the remarkable recoveries of sixty-seven patients as they underwent treatment with this new therapy. I felt compelled to get this information out to others in the medical community who might want to try this therapy, and to the patients who had so much to gain from it.

"I was an independent practicing physician, not associated with a prestigious University or large drug company. The chances of my getting published in a major medical journal were slim. There was very little monetary profit from this therapy that might encourage a drug company to engage in a major research project. "The study was heavily peer reviewed. Over thirty separate universities were involved in the original peer review process, an unheard of number for a journal publication where usually one or two individuals review an article. All of the reviews were positive.

"I needed to get the information out, so I decided to publish the study I had done of all the stroke patients who came to the Institute, and publish it in Lifeline Journal on MedForum.com, an Internet site. That way anyone could read it and learn about this remarkable turn of events.

"The study's point was that major neurological recovery occurred in patients even with previously "permanent" neurological deficits. Furthermore, regardless of the severity of the stroke or length of time since the stroke, most patients improved neurologically when treated with vasodilators using the method outlined in the study.

"All patients with stable neurological deficits after stroke, who came to our Institute and continued with treatments for more than four visits, were included in this study. It was done in 1996 and early 1997.

"Most patients had been without any improvement for more than a year before starting therapy. The patients began no other therapies during the time of the study. The average age was 48; however, the age range was from 25 to 88 years.

"They had neurological improvements, regardless of the size of their strokes or how long ago they had occurred. No patients worsened with the treatment. In the first year, eighty-two percent had enormous recoveries of their lost abilities. Twelve percent had minor improvement and six percent had no apparent improvement. Improvement continued throughout the entire year for patients, but some patients got better more slowly than others. The patient's age didn't matter nor how long ago their stroke occurred.

"Patients in this study removed their braces, got up out of wheelchairs, gained strength, improved their walking, arm movement, and hand dexterity, lost pain, improved their cognition and speech, became more alert, had better balance, and a host of other improvements.

"I have since treated thousands of patients, always refining and improving the therapy. With conventional treatment, about forty percent of all stroke victims suffer another stroke within five years. So far, my patients have not had second strokes.

"Why don't other doctors use this treatment?"

"Their office has to be set up for it. If they don't have all this machinery, they can't do it. It is expensive. I've tried to keep the costs down as much as possible. But to get this kind of breakthrough and have no one listen is very frustrating.

"After I was nominated for the Nobel Prize, physicians were willing to talk about it. I stopped getting the third degree from screening committees for speaking at conventions. The Nobel nomination really helped.

"Now patients are coming from around the country, even around the world. We are changing the paradigms in a grass-roots way. Patients go home and their doctors see the results. Then they are supportive and will spread the word. Our whole process is designed for reassurance. We want to change patients' expectations for their future. Many of them have lost hope and we want to give them back that hope. We want them to continue to expect to get better, because if they expect to improve, they will stick with the treatment and get better. A positive attitude helps.

"We need to change their spouses' views and their caregivers' views. When people have strokes they lose their friends and their social structure. They can't get in and out of bathrooms and can't get to church. They don't get better.

They complain. Hostility and dependency develop. We have to change all that.
"We need support groups that help. A right side stroke patient has different problems from a person who has had a stroke on the left side. There is so much to do and so little time to do it."
I looked at my watch. It was twelve-thirty. Our plane left at three.
Sharon opened the door. "We have a question."
"Just ten minutes more," Dr. Hammesfahr said, but he did stand up.
He had talked intensely and for a long time and he still had more to say. When Dad and I finally stood to go, Dr. Hammesfahr kept on talking as we walked out of the office. His enthusiasm was infectious.
We made an appointment for three months hence. I wanted to shout to the world "You can recover!" What could I do for these people? Whom can I tell about this therapy?
Sharon hugged and kissed us goodbye. Dr. Hammesfahr shook Dad's hand and said, "See you soon Dr. Robinson."
"I'm going to write a book about this therapy," I said almost before I knew it. "That way everyone can know about your work."
"That would be wonderful. If you need help, let me know."
As we left the Institute, Dad burst full-voiced into song.
"Smile, darn you, smile
You know this old world is a great old world after all,
Smile, darn you, smile
And right away watch Lady Luck pay you a call
Things are never dark as they are painted.
It's time for you and Lady Luck to get acquainted.
Make life worthwhile, come on and smile, darn you, smile."

When Dad was young, he could fill a concert hall with his voice, without a microphone. Since the stroke his voice had been weak and tentative. That day it was loud and strong, just like it had been before the stroke. There was another change for me to record.

We made a mad dash for the motel and loaded our bags in the car. I gave Dad lunch so he could take his pills, cleaned out the refrigerator, washed the dishes, paid the bill at the Aloha Motel and drove to the airport. We arrived twenty minutes behind schedule. I returned our little green car and Dad and I checked in and walked to the gate.

It was only then that I realized that Dad had walked all the way on his own. Joy! I'd rolled him out in a wheelchair when we arrived, but he walked into it for our trip home. If we needed proof that he was better, there it was.

"What's this about writing a book?" Dad asked as we settled into our seats.

"I mean it," I said. "I have all of my daily journals and notes from the meetings. I'm going to turn those into the story of our visit with Dr. Hammesfahr."

"Am I going to be in it?" he asked.

"You're the star." I took his hand in mine. "We're partners."

As we neared Chicago, the horizon became a long flat line with yellow fading to pale blue above it. The clouds swallowed us into a whitewater dreamland as we began to descend, falling off the cliff and floating. Each moment was the same and each moment was new. A small event had occurred, and forever after there would be a chasm at that moment between the past and the future.

While each thing we did seemed the same as we what we had done on the way down to the Institute, flying in a plane, looking at the clouds, opening a magazine, all of it was different. Everything had a slightly different color, a slightly different texture, a slightly different smell. Every action had a different meaning. Every thought came with a different expectation. Now we had hope, but it was hope with strings attached. It was hope with a great deal of work to be done. I reached for the airline magazine and paged through it, looking for Dr. Hammesfahr's ad. It was not there. I looked out at the clouds. They were the same.

I have long been interested in paths, whether they were my mother's time worn paths across the sand hills of Nebraska or the serpentine road to understanding myself and others, in which my father had schooled me. When I was in high school I took a world history class from the football coach. It was not a particularly stellar class. We often spent Mondays discussing the game he had coached the weekend before. But he did assign us a major research project that stuck with me over the years. My report was on Taoism. I typed it on my aqua blue Royal Portable with a much-used ribbon that made faint marks on the onionskin paper. The translucent pages whispered mysterious secrets as I turned them.

After I finished writing, I spent a long time drawing the cover, a Chinese letter that symbolized humanity. I did not have a thick pen and so, patiently, I drew tiny thin line after line, putting one small line beside another to blacken the page-sized letter I had chosen. Each fine line contributed to the whole, but took only a small space on the page. Each action was a thin thread that portended the future. I imagined the old Greek crone, Clotho, spinning out my thread of life. It took hours. I didn't know what a Mandala was and had never experienced meditation. I just had a very thin pen point and some extra time.

The memory of that drawing stayed with me for forty years. Like that page, I built my life with infinitesimal actions but no deep understanding. Was all this living supposed to mean something? I meandered, like the Platte River in Nebraska. Mostly, I just went with the flow.

As a teacher, being of service was easy. Taking action in that career was imperative. Becoming self-aware was not easy. I thought I had lived through a multitude of problems and choices, a career, marriage, children, travel, divorce, a late-life love, and now retirement, common experiences for American woman these days. In truth, without being aware of it, I'd chosen a pretty straight path. Now I resolved to undertake to live my life as simply as possible. I wanted to remember how important it was to be able to unfold my fingers to get a manicure or to tie my shoes. I wanted to be happy that I could sleep horizontally in a bed rather than upright in a chair. I wanted to remember to feel thankful that I could move my own body when I rolled over in bed in the morning. I wanted to think of Dorothy's simple wish for her daughter Heather, every time I said, "Hi Steve."

31
I Think I'd Like to Live Now
Wednesday, October 25
Day Twenty-three, Medication Day Twenty

Back at home, I typed "Dad's Improvements" at the top of a page and began a list.

Dad's Improvements:
  (Optimum blood pressure – 135/75)
  PAIN
  - Significantly less pain in both arm and leg
  - Tingling sensations that indicate nerves are being activated again
  - Stopped taking Baclofen for tension in arm

  BRAIN
  - Thinks better
  - Does not search for words
  - Returning vocabulary
  - Maintains ideas until conversations are finished

  VISION
  - Full peripheral vision / back to normal after thirty-three percent loss
  - Improved perception

ARM
- Arm looser and fingers looser
- Can cross his bad arm to opposite side and brush a bug off his shoulder
- Reaches over his head
- Uses his right arm and fingers for some tasks
- Returning sensation in hand and arm

LEG
- Knee bends
- Ankle bends
- Toes bend and wiggle
- More control over his ankle bending
- Walks faster
- Gait is better
- Longer strides
- Easier with steps, no hesitation
- Walks short distances without cane
- Walks in bare feet

ACTS OF DAILY LIVING
- Showers by himself
- Dries his back using both hands
- Shaves himself
- Hits mouth with food when eating, much less messy
- Drinks out of a bottle
- Clearer speech
- Crosses legs (Don't do it!)
- Sleeps less during the day
- More alert
- Holds clever and intellectual conversations (Warning: watch his jokes!)
- Returned sense of smell
- Improved sense of taste
- Sings loudly

Educational psychologist's evaluation after 2½ weeks:
MOTOR SKILLS
- Right hand able to tap 7 times in one minute / previously 0 times in one minute
- Left hand improved from 43 taps to 67 taps in one minute
- Remembered year, month, day, and President / previously knew none of them
- Improved decoding ability
- Improved short-term memory of numbers
- Improved processing of information
- Improved organization of thoughts

Physical Therapist's Evaluation After 3 Weeks:
- Balance improved from 2 seconds to 3 seconds on right foot and 4 seconds to 8 seconds on left foot
- Turns quickly
- Ten steps in 10 seconds on small raised platform alternating legs
- Improved sensation in arm and leg / feels things now
- Stands with one foot in front of the other and balances with a much narrower stance

"This is impressive, Dad," I said, showing him my work. "Look at how long this list is! Can you read it in that eight-point type? I wanted to get it all on one page." It was printed on blue paper so that he could find it easily when he got back to The Fort Armstrong Retirement Home.

"I can read it." He studied it as he slugged down one of his eight glasses of water for the day.

My son, Rollins, took the morning off to come over to see GP, as he calls his grandfather. They were in the kitchen talking while I was trying to organize the last minute medications, meals, and Dad's Blue Binder from Dr. Hammesfahr's office. I rearranged the book so that my sister would have an easy time understanding what had to be done when it got to be her turn later that day. Then I arranged for a van to take Dad home to Rock Island. I called my sister to tell her the pick-up time. I typed more lists, for his doctor, my sister, and the Fort Armstrong Hotel. Finally, the doorbell rang.

"That's the van man! Let's get going, Dad."

Rollins picked up his GP's suitcase and took it down the two flights of stairs and loaded it into the van.

"Take my blood pressure before I go." Dad held out his arm and I slid the machine up and pressed the digital button. It was 119/68. It was little low, under 70. We navigated the two flights of stairs, said our good-byes, and got him settled in the van.

"Let me kiss you good-by." I kissed his sweet smelling cheek. His sweet smelling cheek. It was only three weeks ago that he couldn't smell himself, but all the rest of us could. His last words to me before he left were not the terrifying ones from a month ago, "I'd rather die than live like this." Instead, he said, "I think I'd like to live now."

I closed the door and he waved goodbye. I stood at the curb. Our journey had seemed so long yet it happened so fast. First there was nothing. Then there was a major life-altering change. It was a rushed ending for such a profound event. I wanted there to be a climax for the end. I was left feeling a bit empty.

My take-charge sister was on duty next. In a way I was relieved. It was her mission now. No, it was our mission, but I was confident that she would follow through.

Phase one was done. Now Dad would go on to phase two and get better and better. I had plane tickets waiting to take him back to Clearwater three months down the road, for the continued fine-tuning of his medications. I could finally relax. For me, for now, it was over.

32
Epilogue
Heather

A few weeks later, I had a call from Dorothy. Heather had been in treatment at the Institute for just seven days.
"We've had a breakthrough!" Dorothy said. "Brooks was in the bedroom, bending Heather's legs and he asked her, 'Why don't you do this by yourself, Heather?'
And she did! Seven times in a row. All by herself. Her eyes were twinkling. She knew she had done something special. I can't wait to tell the doctors tomorrow when we go to the Institute."
A week after that, when they asked Heather to move her legs for Dr. Hammesfahr she wouldn't do it. That afternoon at the Education Session she started to move them again, bending her right knee and then her left and trying to get Dr. Hammesfahr's attention. Suddenly, she let out a huge "Aghhrrrrrr." Everyone looked at her. Eyes sparkling, she kept on moving her legs, shamelessly flirting with Dr. Hammesfahr, who stopped the entire meeting to introduce her. Having been involved in dramatics in high school and college, she knew she was creating a sensation and she didn't mind being center stage at all. She understood everyone's applause was for her and responded to it.
A month later Dorothy and Brooks quit smoking, saying, "It will be so much better for Heather and for us."

Heather's alertness improved and she held her head up more frequently and for longer periods of time. She started drinking lots of water and liked it better than any other drink. She was able to get a hairbrush to her head in thirty seconds instead of a minute and a half. She ran the brush through her hair two times, which was something that she had not done before.

Her legs relaxed and her feet fell to the wheelchair foot rests instead of sticking straight out in muscle spasms. Her toes were pink instead of deep purple. They relaxed and were no longer curled tightly into the soles of her feet. She seldom had spasms or seizures.

Heather continued to have slow recovery. She began watching Dorothy working in the kitchen instead of staying glued to the TV, and she focused her eyes more often. She also asserted her personality, especially when she did not like something.

Two years later, Heather stood for the first time. A month later, she was able to stand for ten minutes with help. She held her balance while being helped to shuffle the twelve feet from her room to the living room. She stood by herself in the swimming pool. Her renewed sense of balance was helped by the fact that her knees no longer collapsed. She had control of her swallowing and sipped from a straw on her own. She controlled her own bladder and was no longer incontinent during the day. Heather began to use consonant sounds and form syllables. Her nurse said that she had seven words and said, "No, Dad." But no one else in the family could confirm that. She had a new sense of self which you can see in her eyes.

She has not said, "Hi, Mom."

Yet.

Two and a half years later Heather and her nurse, Louise danced, ballroom style. It was a shuffle but one with rhythm. Heather's mother described a physical therapy technique in which Louise rotated Heather's big toe and that produced movement in her hip, the trunk of her body and her shoulder. Heather could not have done that unless her muscles were relaxed. Louise described Heather as easier to work with than a year ago.

Heather began using faces mounted on Velcro to describe how she felt each morning. She selected one of the squares with a frown or a smile on it and put it beside the day and date that Louise put up each morning.

Her Shaker Heights high school class of 1979 had its twenty-fifth year reunion in July and one of her classmates, Jim Brickman the "Romantic Piano Sensation" played a piano concert that he dedicated to Heather. The class paid the expenses to fly Heather and her family and a nurse in to Cleveland for this fundraiser. Heather was on the stage and her mother said she upstaged Jim Brinkman.

Louise and Heather attended the movies once a week and Heather picked the movies. Louise read her the reviews and Heather indicated that she wanted to see the movie by saying 'Yeah' or 'No.'

She says 'Hi,' but not 'Hi, Mom.'

Yet.

Dr. Edward Woodrow Robinson

During the three months after his treatment as the second circle of Dad's brain damage from the stroke began to repair itself, his pain continued to subside, so that he was able to stop taking the four Ibuprofen daily. He was less dizzy after he stopped taking the Baclofen and his balance improved. His arm did not float around anymore. It hung relaxed by his side. He could roll over in his bed more easily.

A week after returning home he read an entire article from a magazine, and could talk about it. It took him all morning, but previously he had been unable to read any more than a paragraph, and even that took great effort. However, the next day when I asked him about the article he did not remember what it had said. It took several more months before he could retain the information that he read.

I was thrilled when he asked if I would send the manuscript for this book to him so he could read what I had written about our journey. He made comments about my stories and I knew that he remembered what I'd written.

In November, he began going to church with Lia. She told me that he walked easily down the aisle, with his feet close together. He even sang the first verses of the hymns. The minister said, "God whispers in funny corners and you have to listen for him."

Dad said, "I'm listening. I'm listening."

His return to health affected everyone around him. He began doing set up lines for a guy at his dining table who liked to tell jokes. His puns and wisecracks kept everyone laughing. When he left the table after breakfast, lunch, and dinner, he sang his way out of the dining hall. Other residents were surprised at first, but soon they joined in when they knew the song. He sang all the way back to his apartment, bringing the other residents out into the halls, especially the craziest among them, who liked the singing best. He spoke to everyone and was much happier.

He began playing bridge on Saturdays with a group he organized at the Hotel. He had played bridge previously, but the groups met elsewhere and were more difficult to get to, especially in the winter. His good friend, Thea, joined him and giggled and joked her way through many a finesse. He took delight in this small woman with her lavender jogging suits and her sparkling eyes. She teased him and touched him, slapping him on the knee and putting her arm through his when they walked together. Living alone, with no close companion, made this friendship important.

When Dad visited Steve and me in Key West at the end of December, he was not feeling well. His blood pressure was erratic, up at one reading and down at the next one. With the erratic blood pressure came more pain. He said that he hurt when he took a step. I worried a lot and tried the salt water trick, but it didn't work. When he got home, his local doctor found a potassium deficiency. A new pill helped that, but by the time Dad returned to Clearwater in January, his medications badly needed adjustment.

Thea flew to Clearwater with him. She could not fly alone, as she was too spacey and would wander off. Dad kept her headed in the right direction when they changed planes in Atlanta. She spent the time with her daughter in Naples, asking over and over where Dad was.

Dad had to stay in Clearwater two extra weeks because his medications were still not adjusted by the end of the first week. Steve and I could not stay with him because Steve was scheduled to undergo radiation treatments for his prostate cancer. Dad suggested that he stay at The Oaks, an assisted living home near the Institute. With much trepidation we left him there. He got himself over to the Institute on the shuttle van for his daily medicine adjustments. One day, the elevator at The Oaks broke down and he walked up five flights of stairs to get to his apartment. That was an unheard of feat for him three months before.

Thea had to extend her stay with her daughter for two weeks until Dad was ready to go home. He got to the airport by himself and home to Rock Island, escorting the vivacious Thea.

At his grandson, Rollins', wedding in June, seven months after he began medication, Dad got through two full days of festivities without taking any naps. He lifted his right leg when walking and didn't drag his right foot. He began to use his right hand to shake hands again because he could keep his fingers loose so he didn't squeeze too hard.

The retirement hotel started an exercise group that met three times a week. My father, who'd always claimed that his daily exercise was to lift a drink from the table to his lips, joined it. The group did easy exercises for the elderly, but the fact that he was actually doing them was definitely a change in his Activities of Daily Living chart.

Dad dismissed the woman who had come to give him a shower three times a week, saying, "I can do it myself. I don't need her any more." He said he was going to spend the money on a once a week massage that would loosen the tension in his neck and shoulders and straighten out the muscle knots in his right arm and leg.

Gradually, Dad returned to a more normal life where there was hope for the future and joy in his daily living. The prognosis was for more gradual improvement as his blood vessels heal and stop their destructive spasms. Who knows how well he will be in a year or two years or five years?

Dr. Hammesfahr recently tested Steve and me with the Transcranial Doppler (TCD). My TCD on one side was worse than my Dad's. Steve's were better. He put us both on nitroglycerin cream. After using the nitro, I immediately felt my sinus cavities open. Then my shoulders relaxed and I felt calmer. My handwriting improved considerably. I typed faster, with fewer mistakes. Steve's balance improved and he walked with his feet closer together. Maybe I will be rid of the dyslexia I have had all my life. Maybe Steve will be able to ride a bike with me again.

After a season of renting, we bought a condo in Key West. It was totally empty. The floors and walls were white. I watched the sun rise each morning over the Atlantic Ocean. The winds ruffled though the palm fronds and the empty rooms. The feng shui dragons were happy. The future may be unknown, but it was not bleak, it was beckoning.

Oh, yes, one more thing. Dad got his whistle back.

One year later

Thea went into the hospital for minor surgery on hemorrhoids and died on the operating table. My father was devastated, angry and bitter. Crushed and terrified at the same time, he accused the hospital of killing her.

Shortly after that he was diagnosed with a carcino-sarcoma, a very aggressive cancer. He refused surgery, saying that surgery killed Thea. He was treated with radiation and chemotherapy. His doctor told him to get his affairs in order as he had only a few months to live. He had hope that he could overcome the cancer as he had overcome the stroke.

December 18, two years, three months later my father died.

Dad lasted much longer than doctors expected. His gentle strength and hope for the future sustained him. He kept his newly found ability to think, speak and remember until the end. During the last month of his life he was under twenty-four hour hospice care at my sister's home. He refused the morphine that they offered him until the last three days of his life because he didn't want to be "out of it," when he met Rollins' son, his new great grandson.

During his last month, he counseled two of the regular hospice aides, one with teenage daughter problems and the other with a philandering husband and an intense desire to go to nursing school. One of his final acts was to write a check to her for first semester's tuition to return to school. He died with grace in the home of my sister at four AM. His adopted son was seated next to him.

A week after he died, he and mother visited me in a dream. I told them that I was glad that they had found each other since they had loved each other so much in life. Dad said, "It's not like that here, Robin." I took it to mean that there was a broader definition of love after death. Mother added, "But we want you to know that we both love you very much." Then they left. I still think that mother talks to me through the birds and I have discovered that Dad sends me messages through the songs that pop into my head. They both are very much a part of my life.

Afterward

Dr. Hammesfahr was nominated for the Nobel Prize in Medicine and Physiology in 1999 for advances in Stroke and Brain Injury. The nomination was of the highest order, a congressional nomination from the Chairman of the Subcommittee on Health and Environment, Michael Bilirakis, who was also in charge of Medicare at the time. It was for the work he started in 1994. It was one of one hundred and thirty six worldwide nominations and was posted as recommended reading on the Nobel Prize web site at the Karolinski Institute Web Site.

His article, "Reversing Stroke Using Common Vasodilators" can be found on the Worldbook Medical Encyclopaedia Web Site.

He applied for a medical patent in the summer of 2001. After a five-year investigation, the U.S. Patent Office issued a patent on the therapy, citing its novelty and effectiveness. It was the first United States patent in history granted for the treatment of neurological diseases including severe migraines, seizures, coma, stroke, brain injury, cerebral palsy, hypoxic injuries and other neuro-vascular disorders with medications that restore blood flow to the brain. The therapy was extended to treat disabilities such as ADD, ADHD, Dyslexia, Tourette's and Autism as well as behaviorally and emotionally disturbed children with great success.

As with anyone with a new idea, especially one that challenges the very basis of the field of neurology, Dr. Hammesfahr had a difficult a road to travel as he developed this remarkable discovery.

Medicare questioned the use of the Ultrasound as a monitoring device and stopped paying for patient's treatment. Losing Medicare coverage for patients was a huge obstacle. As he could not believe that Medicare had stopped payment permanently, he continued to treat his Medicare patients free of charge. After six months of this he was forced to begin charging patients. He was upset that the therapy was only available to those who had the money to pay for it and that it was denied to the people who did not have those resources.

After seven years of investigation, an internal Medicare review identified that the treatment is new, successful and works to restore function in patients even with long term 'permanent' injuries from stroke and brain injury. Payment was approved.

However, for the related disorders that Dr. Hammesfahr discovered also had a vascular basis, like learning disabilities, epilepsy and seizures, autism, dementia, memory loss, and so on, it took an additional two years and a federal administrative law judge to review the evidence, the patient files, and to order Medicare to pay for the treatment of these conditions with Dr. Hammesfahr's therapy. Thirty separate, almost identical decisions were written, identifying these other conditions for the first time in history, as being in part vascular and treatable with Dr. Hammesfahr's vascular protocol. They also, again, confirmed that the treatment was effective in what had been considered to be permanent stroke and brain injuries.

Medicare officials issued a report calling Dr. Hammesfahr's therapy "medically reasonable and necessary." They resumed patient coverage of payments. Private insurance companies followed suit. Unlike when my father was being treated, now, Medicare, Medicaid and other insurances are routinely accepted.

The Florida Board of Medicine dismissed a suit against his therapy after investigation. Judge Susan Kirkland said that he was "the first physician to treat patients successfully to restore deficits caused by stroke." This determination was upheld by a full vote of the Florida Board of Medicine in 2002.

The federal government has recognized Dr. Hammesfahr's clinical expertise, naming him Reviewer and Chief Reviewer for evaluation and funding for new clinical research programs. He has also been a court-recognized expert and a court-ordered treating physician for these techniques that he pioneered. He has lectured and published extensively.

Doctors are often suspicious of new therapies, particularly those that depart from the norm, or from the conventional wisdom, and can be quick to label them baseless and unscientific. What he was doing from the beginning, far from being unscientific, involved the most careful and sophisticated use of the most sophisticated equipment and the optimum application of the newest techniques and medications. Despite this he still had major problems from the skeptical world of disbelievers.

Dr. Hammesfahr will consult with and share his methodology with any physician anywhere in the world and is delighted to work with local physicians wherever a patient lives. He hopes that the doctors will take the time to understand what the Institute is doing in order to follow through with care, at least monthly, between the patient's visits to the Institute. Keeping a patient on the right dosage despite varying weather conditions and personal activities is important. Having the doctor from the patient's home town on board is vital to the patient's well being. Most physicians respond well when their patients return home and they can see the changes that have occurred. All patients need is an open-minded and receptive doctor at home.

He and his colleagues continue to treat patients at the Hammesfahr Neurological Institute. The Institute's phone number is 1-800 673-6400. For more information visit the Institute's informative web site at www.hnionline.com.

Acknowledgments from the Author

For their help in the creation of this book I am grateful to:

Betty Sitbon, the perceptive artist who encouraged me to keep a journal of this experience.

My sister, who allowed me to use her as the conflict without getting angry.

Judith Buckner who gave me encouragement, hope and her good editing.

Esme Raji Codell, a student who exceeds her teacher, for her encouragement and good publishing advice.

Gloria Asbel, Maureen Breen and Joan Martorelli for their sharp proofreading eyes.

M. Anne and Dick Vick, who read aloud to my stroke damaged mother and taught me the importance of friendship.

Nancy Butler-Ross, Bonnie Doerr, and Donna Smith for great listening and excellent advice.

Steven Breslau, for holding me together when I had too much to do.

The entire staff at the Hammesfahr Neurological Institute whose good humor and positive attitudes gave us joy on our trip to recovery.

Dr. William Hammesfahr, whose brilliant, observant mind made *Peeling the Onion: Reversing the Ravages of Stroke* possible.

To my mother, who died too soon.

And above all, my father, who taught me empathy and understanding.

Acknowledgements from Dr. Hammesfahr

Over the last ten years, I have counted over one hundred and fifty professionals who were involved in taking the discovery of our initial day's observations and turning them into a safe and successful therapy. I am grateful to them for their commitment. Their commitment gave me courage.

I would like to add to the names mentioned in the book, Jacques Fortin, MD, physiatrist, counselor, and friend, who worked long hours in the early years. Dr. Michael Eastridge, whose detailed work extended the understanding of blood flow, learning, and personality. Donald Adkins, registered EEG technician, and one of the fathers of EEG work in this country, whose tireless efforts and concentration aided my understanding of the recovery process and the drug interactions in these patients.

I would like to honor patients, like Ron Clarke, Billy and Pat and many others who, after recovering, volunteered their time, feedback, and observations to help other patients keep their spirits up and recover.

I thank the journalists who have tried to share the good news and get other physicians to incorporate this treatment by raising their awareness of it. They weathered the repercussions of attacks on their credibility, and still fought on to give people knowledge and a second chance.

There is so much for which to thank my parents and my brothers, that I couldn't begin a list.

Most of all, I thank my wife and children. The personal and financial stress of going a new way can't be understood except by those who have walked that path. Without my wife, Gina, and my children, Alanna and Austin, who gave me strength, I don't think that this therapy would have survived. They supported me even when they were scared, tired, or stressed.

And, I thank Woody, whom I loved and will carry in my heart forever.

Disclaimer

This book is a trip though the emotions of a patient and caregiver. It is not a medical prescription for individuals, as the process of evaluating patients is very individualized and needs to be done in a controlled medical environment. This story is creative non-fiction. It is seen through my eyes and memory. While I have retained the names of the staff at the Hammesfahr Neurological Institute, I have changed the names of the patients and other medical personnel. Any inaccuracies in the book are entirely mine and do not reflect on the Hammesfahr Neurological Institute.

Robin Robinson

QUICK ORDER FORM
Peeling the Onion:
Reversing the Ravages of Stroke

Website: www.sorapublishing.com
Email Orders: sorapublishing@comcast.net
Postal orders: Send this form

Name: _____

Address: _____

City: _____**State:** _____ **Zip** _____

Telephone: _____

Email Address: _____

Price: $19.95
Sales Tax: Please add $1.50 if shipped to Florida.
Shipping and Handling:
U.S.: $4.05 for first book and $2.00 for each additional book
International: $9.00 for first book; $5.00 for each additional book (estimate).

PAYMENT BY CHECK OR MONEY ORDER
SORA Publishing
Robin Robinson
1800 Atlantic Boulevard, A-405
Key West, Florida 33040